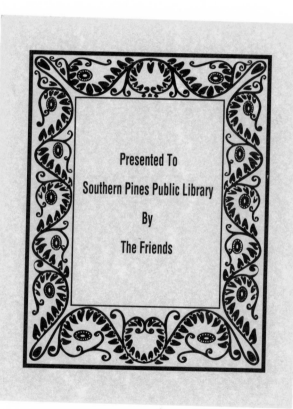

I'm Not As Old As I Used to Be

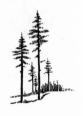

Also by Frances Weaver
in Large Print:

The Girls with the Grandmother Faces

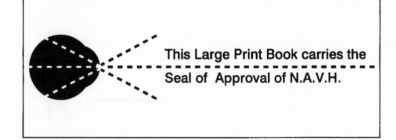

This Large Print Book carries the
Seal of Approval of N.A.V.H.

I'm Not As Old As I Used to Be

Reclaiming Your Life
in the Second Half

FRANCES WEAVER

*With Incidental Drawings from the
Author's Sketchbook*

Thorndike Press • Thorndike, Maine

Published in 1997 by arrangement with Hyperion.

Thorndike Large Print ® Basic Series.

The tree indicium is a trademark of Thorndike Press.

The text of this Large Print edition is unabridged.
Other aspects of the book may vary from the original edition.

Set in 16 pt. Plantin by Minnie B. Raven.

Printed in the United States on permanent paper.

Library of Congress Cataloging in Publication Data

Weaver, Frances.
    I'm not as old as I used to be : reclaiming your life in the
second half / Frances Weaver ; with incidental drawings
from the author's sketchbook.
      p. cm.
    Large print ed.
    Originally published : New York : Hyperion, 1997.
    ISBN 0-7862-1248-9 (lg. print : hc : alk. paper)
    1. Weaver, Frances. 2. Aged women — United States —
Biography. 3. Self-realization in old age — United States.
4. Grief. I. Title.
[HQ1064.U5W394 1997b]
305.26′092—dc21
[B]   97-36712

*For my daughter, Allison,
who just turned 50.*

Contents

Introduction   9

Chapter One: I Feel Like I'm
   Still Me   13

Chapter Two: Getting Tired —
   Getting Old   21

Chapter Three: Oh, But You're
   Not a <u>Real</u> One!   30

Chapter Four: The Remembrance
   Is Grievous unto Us   36

Chapter Five: Facing Life Alone   44

Chapter Six: Grief — Write It Out!   48

Chapter Seven: Downhill Slide   63

Chapter Eight: A Little Learning
   Goes a Long Way   74

Chapter Nine: What Shall I Do Now?   91

Chapter Ten: How in the World?   111

Chapter Eleven: Elsewhere 126

Chapter Twelve: Publishing? You? 136

Chapter Thirteen: Granny! How
 You've Changed! 176

Chapter Fourteen: Today,
 a Different World 188

Chapter Fifteen: Hang onto
 the Rapture 194

Epilogue: Welcome to the Club! 201

Introduction

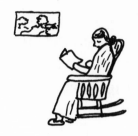

Getting old — really old — cannot in any way be called easy. Life, in our periods of change and adjustment, does not flow like a meandering brook through a lush pasture. A more suitable comparison to the creek in the "wash" behind Granddad's house comes to my mind. Some days it flows gently. Other days the water gushes through, making ruts along its path. Still other times the entire stream disappears and hope goes with it. But not for long.

Conversation with one of my older cousins reminded me of this. Change in our lives causes problems. Going to kindergarten, starting junior high, getting married, becoming a parent, looking for a job — all of these carry some trauma. No person, particularly a widow in her seventies, will try to tell you that getting old makes life more pleasant *all* of the time.

This book and my own ideas carry only one message: We have it within ourselves to create a simpler, more productive, less stressful way of life that will make us more interesting to ourselves and our families without getting in anyone else's way and without expecting service and sympathy at every turn.

No, it will not happen overnight, nor by the flick of a dial, but the effort pays dividends in unthought-of ways. Surprise yourself!

Jitterbug Rap

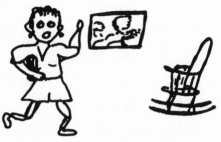

*(A steady beat on the coffee table or the arm
of your chair will help as you read this.)*

Come on you Grannies, get in the groove
This old folks' world is startin' to move
No more waitin' for the phone to ring
No more huntin' for blues to sing
You and I got plenty to do
Just playin' catch-up will take a few
Months of practice then we'll really swing
Just like Benny or some Dorsey thing.
The more we sit, the more we grumble
You'll feel like your hind end's caught in
the rumble
Seat of your boyfriend's old Model A
Back in the thirties — that'd be the day.
Forget about the old days? Not if
you're smartest
You can make new days — you're a
new-day artist

Take all the good stuff you know how
to do
Match it up easy with somethin' brand
new.
Surprise all the young bucks, enlighten
your kids
Show you've learned more than
preemptive bids.
Join a few classes, shake those tired limbs
Go for a workout in broken-down gyms
You'll fit right in there if you don't watch
your step
"Fit" is the right word if you're gonna
be hep.
Try a new hobby, tie a new fly
Climb a small mountain just fifty feet high
But get out and do it, don't sit there
and rust
Read a new book, help the old lady dust
Walk at your leisure around the
school track
Then wait a few days before you try to
go back
Don't whine about Dentugrip, Maalox
and Tums
Call up your old cronies — those
lazy bums
Sprawled 'front of TV rotting away
While you're out there having a
wonderful day.

Chapter One

I Feel Like I'm Still Me

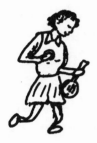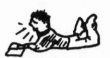

"When I look in the mirror, I just can't believe I'm seeing myself. The face has wrinkles deep as Salt Creek, a saggy neck — I just can't think I've gotten that old. Inside I feel like I always have — the same me. But I surely don't look the same." This lively woman shrugged her shoulders. "Then I make the mistake of looking in a magnifying mirror and I have to go lie down for a while."

She laughed. "I'm eighty now. I guess I should expect that."

I laughed right along with her, but silently admired this old lady for her ability to see herself as she actually appears: an older woman unafraid of admitting her age. We all know women of this sort — admirable women who face the aging process as just one more stage of life, a normal progression of events.

Another friend my age laughed, telling me about her grandson admiring her in her new tennis outfit. "But, Grandma, somebody's let the air out of your arms."

Why not laugh? All sorts of plastic surgery might fool us for a while, but acceptance of our real age, our real stage of life, always shows up on our arms, doesn't it?

I told that arms story to an audience in Vermont. They laughed readily, but one woman approached me later. "One of my grandkids made a remark like that about my arms, and I popped right back at him. I said, oh, can't you do that? That's a trick I learned, and I shook my arms at him. The kid spent the rest of the afternoon out in the yard teaching his neighborhood pals how to do his grandma's arm jiggle."

How different these women and their attitude about aging strikes us when we have been subjected to some of the weepers and whiners of our generation or when we ourselves have felt uncomfortable in the over-the-hill gang for a while. For reasons completely unknown to me, some people resist old age like the plague. You know some of them. So do I. We try to avoid confrontations with these negative oldsters, mostly because we have heard their complaints so often already.

14

Therein lies one of the reasons for avoidance of older folks by younger friends and family and more often by their peers. The stereotype of the older man or woman with nothing positive to say has a firm foundation in the conversations of these old codgers who spend every waking moment (it seems) looking for something else to fret about. Any weather causes arthritis to act up. Any hairdresser doesn't know how to give a decent shampoo. Any bank teller talks snippy. Any music sounds like loud trash. Any skirts are too short or too long. Any TV show should be banned from the air. Any supermarket has a rotten arrangement of their produce. You know. You have heard it all as often as I have. Most of all, these people resent any reminder of their advanced age without "due respect."

One of the funniest stories, told to me with a grim face by a fancy lady in a fancy place in California, concerned another very fancy lady in a French bakery, also fancy. The woman had picked up her advance order for some wondrous pastries, only to be delayed by a beagle-voiced clerk who fairly shouted, "Say, aren't you a senior citizen?"

The astonished customer said, softly, "Yes, I suppose I am."

"Well," bellowed the clerk, "you get a free cookie!"

15

That shop lost a customer that day. The woman stomped out of the store with her cookie, looking sour. Insulted and angry, she vowed never to return.

I often wonder about such reactions. All of our lives follow a certain pattern. We know that from the time we know anything. Some people are young, some are older. Some have blonde or brown hair, some have gray. Some kids are big enough to drive cars, others ride bikes. The big kids in the schoolyard swing on the big swings. Some women have children, some have grandchildren, too. Some people rollerskate or hike in the mountains, others say they're "past that."

Avoiding old age, or trying to, makes as much sense as avoiding puberty. There it comes, ready or not. The behavioral scientists have pontificated for years. Old age can be handled. I love the quote from B. F. Skinner in his book, *Enjoy Old Age*: ". . . we suggest ways of changing the world of old people so that they can do more of the things they *want* to do and will more often *like* whatever they do." A comforting thought, but largely ignored by the age-resistant group I run into in the supermarket. Basically, some of the older people I know act as if they expected to be thirty-five forever.

They say things like, "You'll never get me on a bus with a lot of old fogies," or words to that effect. More often than not they are the gals with the jet-black hair in the June Allyson pageboy, wearing the same bright red lipstick we loved in college.

Jane Porcino in *Growing Older, Getting Better* writes, "The resourcefulness of women seems to increase as they age." Of course it does, Jane. We didn't just fall off the turnip truck. Older woman have found ways to cope, to recycle, to make do, to invent, to screen possibilities, and to face reality. The problem I see now comes from the reluctance of so many older women to understand and appreciate that fact in their own lives as the years roll by. Now that we have time to think for and about ourselves, creativity builds on past experience. Like the woman I met who started an entire new phase of her life by making bibs out of wash cloths. She didn't fret about what the neighbors thought about her going to craft fairs "with the other old goats."

One of my favorite lecture stories came from a preacher's wife in Florida, where old-folks jokes abound. She told me about a fine gentleman named George. George could be counted on in the community for every sort of good work. He helped with the poor, he visited the sick, he served his church, he never missed a Rotary meeting without making up in the next town. Everyone in town admired George and knew that his generosity and his kindness could be counted on.

But George had one hang-up: He did not want to look old. When George noticed how his spreading waistline added years to his looks, he joined a gym. That made him feel better. At the same time, a definite baldness distressed him when he looked in the mirror to admire his flattened girth. Off went George to a hair store where a sweet young thing convinced him that a hairpiece took twenty years off his age.

Well, George left that store feeling like a million bucks. He concentrated so much on his new youthful appearance that he ignored the traffic. George stepped off the curb just in time to be knocked down by a big truck coming around the corner. Flat on his back with his new hairpiece askew, George shouted his displeasure:

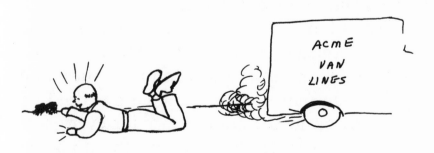

"God! How could You let this happen to me? I've spent my whole life doing good for others! I've tried in every way to be the right kind of a person! And now You let this big truck run me down!"

A voice thundered out of the sky. "George! I didn't recognize you!"

We can assume that George understood the message. Compared with what we do or how we contribute to the lives of others, a spreading waistline or receding hairline means less all the time.

Understanding the message of old age doesn't mean giving up or giving in to those fellow-agers who constantly ask, "You're going to do *what?* At *your* age?" Once we let the reality seep in, saying, "Okay, so I'm older. So what difference does that make?" we can make an honest assessment of ourselves. Instead of a page headed "I'm too old to . . . ," try one marked "Now that I'm older I can . . ."

List the advantages, starting with:

- more leisure time

- fewer family responsibilities now that your children have their own families to fuss about

- a renewed sense of the joy of learning, and more opportunities than ever for continuing education

- freedom from the schedules and routines of a growing family

- more older friends with leisure time

- more labor-saving devices than any generation before us has enjoyed

- a wider range of entertainment

- a greater appreciation of the great outdoors, particularly in this day and age!

A list like this — with the dozens of thoughts you can add to it — makes accepting the fact of being older much more appealing. This age is an integral, expected time of our lives.

Chapter Two

Getting Tired — Getting Old

When does old age start? Does the first gray hair, the first grandchild, the first flight using senior coupons, the first comment about "how young you look" signal the onset of the declining years? Or might that first pair of bifocals mark the transition? The shrinking print in the phone book or the newspaper, the difficulty in hearing the doorbell ring, the tendency to hold onto the rail on steep stairways — all alert us to the aging process.

Others age by the numbers. They seem to think that keeping their age a secret will make those years go away. By and large, most of society regards fifty or fifty-five as the gateway to "advanced maturity," or whatever euphemism they choose to express the unspeakable: We either get old or we die. No other choices. Fifty marks the onset of the golden years for many of us, although few enter this phase in a golden mood.

My fiftieth birthday bothered me very little, but the early fifties drove me just a little crazy. Nowadays the younger generation, our offspring, make a big deal out of the "Big 0" birthdays, as if the millennium had arrived. They outdo each other with grand parties or funny jokes. The people I knew did not carry on so about another year gone by. My fiftieth birthday went practically unnoticed. A couple of years passed before I felt the twinge of approaching old age.

One summer morning marked the turning point when I started to consider my age seriously. On most mornings my hypercompulsive surgeon husband would leap out of bed before I managed to disentangle myself from the sheets. Just once I was up and dressing before he made the big dash for the shower. Not our usual pattern. He lounged there in the bed watching me dress.

"You know," he commented, "I see women in my office all day long without their clothes on. You are the best-looking fifty-three-year-old woman I have ever seen."

What a nice compliment. How did I respond? Did I smile and thank him? Kiss him on the forehead? Jump back in the bed? No. I turned on him like a cat with its tail in the wringer and hollered, "Listen, Buster, *you're* fifty-three; *I'm* fifty-two!"

Later that same day I went across the road (we lived in the mountain community of Beulah, Colorado, then) to visit our aging neighbors. Judge and Mrs. Calahan had arrived for the summer from Garden City, Kansas. After warm greetings and all of the expected comments and questions, Mrs. Calahan took on an air of apology. "I hope you'll excuse the judge for not greeting you. He's napping. Lately he needs a little sleep every afternoon. His age, you know. You see, he's eighty-two and I'm not eighty yet."

Walking back to our house, recalling the way I had jumped on John about our age difference when he tried to be complimentary, it occurred to me: I just might spend the next thirty years harping about that minuscule fact. As he got out of his car in the front drive that evening, I apologized for my inappropriate response to his flattery, but after that, somehow I felt older. Like we had joined the Geritol crowd.

That "old feeling," not at all like the one we sang about back in the thirties, hung around in the back of my head for quite a while. Not full-blown depression, just an awareness of how much younger some of my friends seemed to look, for example. I found a new hairdresser, had my "colors done." I noticed and envied those other mothers whose entire swarm of children went to second or third grade while my youngest graduated from high school. John's creeping baldness showed up more each day. Reaching for the good dishes on the upper shelves made me think about aspirin. No doubt about it. Old age had caught me in one swoop.

I slowed down. After all, a woman my age had to take life a little easier. I might break a hip or develop varicose veins. Younger women could take my altar duty or chair the committees. No sense staying involved in so many activities. Old women didn't do that. Most of the old women, I had noticed, spent their time getting older.

Getting older took up most of my time for a while. Looking back over the past twenty years, the truth finally surfaced: The old rockin' chair had gotten me not because of age; I was tired.

Tired? Of what? Of living the fairly comfortable life of a surgeon's wife? Of having a fine home in the mountains? Of four youngsters now grown and in pretty good shape?

No. I had worn myself and my ambitions

out with a lifestyle both demanding and rewarding, but in terms of other people. This pattern applied to most women my age, I've discovered. Going back over the years, I see now how that aging mentality crept up on me. After all, I had followed the expected path for my generation, and that had exhausted my energy and my interest.

All of us, those newly married in the bloom of those postwar years, had families as soon as we could. After all, we had waited through and survived the war. Young mothers on our block typified the ambitious, enthusiastic women of our generation. We did everything. We started libraries in our new community and took our kids to every lesson known to man or beast at that time. We gloried in our great Prairie School in suburban Kansas City and served willingly as room mothers and scout leaders.

"A drop of O'Cedar behind each ear and a cut onion in the hot oven" covered our tracks. We watched each others' children, car-pooled, taught Sunday school, visited the grandparents regularly, just as most young mothers did in the fifties. We discussed Dr. Spock and convinced each other we were good parents.

Our social lives grew door-to-door or from

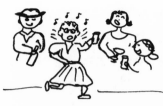one backyard to another. Nobody had time or money for grand cocktail parties or big Saturday nights on the town.

That aspect of our lives changed considerably as our husbands completed medical training, law school, or beginning jobs of all sorts. The years of partying and drinking began in our early thirties. We added new excitement to already overcrowded schedules by discovering the relaxation and release of tension (therefore the great "value") of occasional drinking. What began as one or two drinks at a party soon became drinking with some regularity.

But most of all, we, as women, worked hard at doing and being almost everything to our families and our community. Comparing notes on those early family days, I am convinced my energetic cover-all-the-bases outlook on life differed little from the others of those years.

What time I had for myself went into taking part in the Service League and the church, with a little Republican stuff thrown in. Every cause west of any given point had a committee, a fund raiser, a project worthy of the attention of any housewife who made her home and family her career. The working mothers faced even greater demands.

You would have a hard time naming any cause I haven't been active in. From the medical auxiliary (selling *Today's Health* magazines) to the altar guild and the precinct caucus, I did it all. That made me think I amounted to something aside from the expected wife and mother. How well I filled any or all of those roles I'd rather not say. My lifestyle could be described as "busy" if not actually contributing any value to our world. I had so many outside interests for my own "fulfillment" that John told some of our friends, "Frances thinks she has to have a foot on every ice floe that goes by." True? Perhaps.

No wonder I felt tired and old when my fifties arrived. I had been pushing myself through all sorts of organizations and responsibilities for years. My friends did that, too. The women who took a less active part in community affairs, who did not entertain regularly, who refused to work on the Heart Fund or the Cancer Drive, failed the Good Wife, Good Mother Test. Far be it from me to join *that* crowd.

Thus it happened, when John's sweet comment about my good looks in my fifties brought me up short, that I felt life fading away and the past overwhelming me as I faced these years. My sense of worthwhileness had for years hinged on whatever I did for the children, my home and husband, and all those good causes, as well as pacifying my mother. Suddenly I felt (I realize now) that the causes could survive without my chairmanship, the children had grown to adulthood in spite of my mistakes in mothering, and I could grow up myself, as far as my mother was concerned. I sat around more, went out for lunch more, partied more, drank more, ate more, gossiped more, and fretted more about fewer important things than I had in my busy life.

This describes accurately my state of mind — the state of my life — in my early fifties. Partial rescue or reform — today we'd say "recycling" — began with the kite-flying group about which I have written volumes. Basically, kite-flying with other women my age opened the way to understanding the less-structured life we faced in our "golden years." Our activities had served as an identity. We qualified as den mothers, altar-guild workers, hospital volunteers — all of which brought some recognition. Now we began to think of ourselves in a different light. I had not realized that these girls felt as I did.

The most drastic, compelling recycle in

my life cannot be ignored or swept under the rug in telling this story, however. John's sudden death at fifty-five precipitated my taking a long hard look at myself. Just how do you intend to go on living as you have, dependent on "making the good times roll," now that you're forced to rely on yourself? I asked that question gazing into the mirror. Only one answer came back: I had to stop drinking.

Alcohol had been a problem I'd ignored or denied for years. (I drank only on special occasions, such as days ending in "y.") Now a widow, a "senior single," I was in full charge of me — nobody to make excuses or take the blame. Obvious. Also obvious: A fairly intelligent woman ought to be able to cope, to control this blight on her life. What I needed most was reliability, the confidence of being able to rely upon myself. Through the help of family and friends, I found my way to sobriety. Without that biggest step in my life, none of the rest of these wonderful years would have happened.

Chapter Three

Oh, But You're Not a Real One!

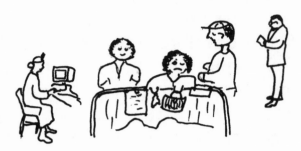

"Franny, dear, you're just grieving because you lost John. That's why you're in this . . . state. You'll be all right when you get over —" Mother stood at the end of my hospital bed, very close to tears. My pure-as-the-driven-snow, strong-drink-will-never-touch-my-lips, drinkers-always-go-to-hell Mother clutching the end of the bed reminded me of the thousands of times I had heard her express those opinions. But now she spoke only to me.

"It's your grief," she repeated.

"No, Mother," I tried to explain again. "John died months ago. That's not the reason I'm here. I have come to this hospital to dry out — to make sure I have help and care if I go into DTs or something. I am an alcoholic."

"Oh," she began to sob, "but you're not a *real* one!"

I wanted to laugh and cry for my mother at the same time. She would rather admit that one of her daughters had almost any problem other than being a drunk. How could I fit her definition of a drunk? As far as she knew, I had never lain in the gutter on Union Avenue or been caught as a hit-and-run driver. After all, she had told us again and again about the evils of drink. How could one of her own daughters be calling herself an alcoholic? And right there in front of people Mother didn't even know.

Mother diagnosed correctly on one count. Grief did have a lot to do with the present crisis. Since John's death, my closest friend and confessor had been Jack Daniels. Jack and I had become inseparable. I depended on him. He responded by pulling a heavy curtain around anything I did not want to see.

I knew about grieving. I knew a lot about everything in those days. I had encountered widows at the supermarket who took up my valuable time showing me wrinkled snap-shots of their dead husbands. I listened, not without irritation, to repetitious tales of the saintly men who had been married to these boring women. My own definition of griev-ing, verified by the whiners, complimented neither these forlorn women nor their departed spouses. That caustic definition does not bear repeating here.

My retreat into consolation from a bottle over sixteen years ago came as naturally as the January winds blowing cold across the Beulah Valley. Addiction to alcohol had been a secret part of my life for years, growing steadily. Actually, it seems almost everyone who knew me knew my secret.

Over the years more and more of my friends had become aware of my telling the same stories, laughing at the same jokes, during an evening when Jack (Daniels) and I were the stars of the show. Telephone conversations after 5:00 P.M. were never remembered the next day. My mood could go from playful to belligerent in a matter of seconds. Time and again I promised myself and my family that this behavior would never happen again, but the next day at 5:00 — well, it was always 5:00 somewhere. . . .

Well-meaning friends gave me books about grieving. They invited me to group sessions. Counseling by professionals bounced off my list of intended activities. Instead, I ate lunch only where drinks were served, socialized only with the "smart" crowd who drank, bought booze from several different stores so no clerk would suspect this splendid, admirable, community-leader doctor's wife of alcoholism. Actually, I had fooled only myself for years.

Then, a few weeks before that day in the hospital, my world started crashing in around me. The grown children and their families who lived close to me found other pastimes on Sunday afternoons. When I invited grandchildren for mountain weekends they suddenly joined teams or had homework. My bridge partners adopted a cool attitude (maybe because I always bid to be the dummy so I could sneak to the kitchen for another drink).

Did I grieve? Not really. I called it grieving when I caught myself listening for John's car in the drive (and poured another to drown my sorrow). I hated going to bed alone, so I took a shot with me. When I had bolstered my courage enough I wrote long-overdue thank-you notes. I tried to write more articles but felt blocked and told myself that was grief. And — this strikes me as most important, looking back — I spent a lot of time going over and over the hurtful times of our marriage. When I got to that stage, resentment raged all out of proportion to the good times.

Gradually, months later (I'm ashamed to say), I recalled the words of Father Hotaling in Concordia, Kansas, after the death of

John's father. Few family members were left. Gathered at the old home place, they drank and reminisced incessantly. In the midst of this, Father Hotaling explained the dangers of drinking too much on such occasions. "When you dull your senses and responses to the reality of the death of a loved one, you obliterate the natural grieving process. If you do not face these occasions with your whole mind, you never recover from the grief and anguish of the dying." At least, he said words to that effect.

Thus, after I had disgraced myself one more time at one more party, it finally dawned on me: My drinking was not saving me, it was killing me. At least, it was killing the me I wanted to be, the me I could depend on. So with family support and help, I went through detox and found a program for sobriety that works for me.

One worry plagued me as I struggled toward a sober life. Would I have any friends if I didn't drink? Would I be popular? Invited out? My social life had great importance. Could I have a sober social life?

Soon after I felt relatively secure while not drinking I went to a party with the old crowd. Halfway through the evening one of my drinking buddies stumbled over to me and fairly shouted, "You know, when you're not drinkin' you're not funny." A sudden ray of brightest light hit me. "You know," I replied, "When I'm not drinking, *you're* not funny."

That one discovery not only paved the way to sobriety, it smoothed the pathway to a productive life without John.

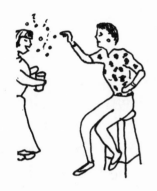

Chapter Four

The Remembrance Is Grievous unto Us

As I sobered up and looked the world squarely in the face, I realized what grieving should be. Primarily, grieving varies from one individual and one family to the next. Attitudes about life itself coupled with the relationship we had with the deceased make a tremendous difference in the manner in which we accept the fact of death. (This might make you angry, but read on, please!) Since grief has become a cause for therapy and hundreds of books, some folks feel almost apologetic in recognizing death as the end of every life at one time or another. I have often said we grieve for ourselves, not for the person who will no longer have to cart that oxygen tank around or live in constant fear of another heart attack or the spread of cancer.

A young man blushed when he admitted

to me, "I cried more when my dog died than when my dad did." Of course he did. The dog had stuck by him through thick and thin, but this particular fellow had never gotten along very well with his demanding, overzealous father. Should he feel guilt? You decide.

We all need, however, to adjust our lives to the change of the cast of characters in our own little drama. We need to get a grip, as the kids say. Good solid advice abounds without descending into the depths of maudlin self-pity. But the best advice remains: Do what suits you, and get on with the rest of your life. Your family will applaud you, your friends will thank you, your neighbors will admire you, and your deceased loved one will be proud of you.

One book in particular, *How to Survive the Loss of a Love* by Melba Colgrove, outlines survival tactics:

Recovering from a loss takes place in three distinct — yet overlapping — stages. They are:

shock/denial/numbness

fear/anger/depression

understanding/acceptance/moving on

Each stage of recovery is:

necessary

natural

a part of the healing process.

The book has been around for twenty years, but the gist of that message still holds true. I had staggered through the denial and numbness to the fear and depression before the truth hit me between the eyes.

These sentiments echoed exactly the feelings of a great many women I've met who felt abandoned, deserted by the husband who had died. I know some men feel the same way about their wives, who they had expected would outlive them. This lost sensation overwhelms a lot of widows to the point that remarriage becomes (to them) the only way out of the misery of living without a mate.

Sociologists and behavioral scientists can undoubtedly pontificate for hours about the degree of self-worth or self-confidence of persons who need marriage. Doesn't it seem to you that some people depend more on a steady, devoted, committed relationship than do others? For these folks, grieving takes the form of finding a replacement for the missing mate.

For most men, this does not present a problem.

In today's world, however, replacement husbands do not regularly appear on every street corner or in every supermarket parking lot waiting for some bereaved soul to claim them. We all realize that we women far outnumber the men of our generation. This means that a new husband, if you connect with one, can be one of life's greatest blessings — but we're all better off not counting on remarriage as the only way to improve our lives. If he shows up, Honey, and he turns out to be the answer to your prayers, more power to you. But not having a husband does not entitle you to waste the rest of your natural life complaining, whining, and waiting for the kids to call.

A positive, progressive grieving period in every life brings the remaining years into focus. Blinding ourselves to the reality of the changes wrought in the lives of the survivors can cripple us almost as much as if we, too, had ceased to live. So, aside from husband-hunting, what can we do to achieve the serenity of life that's possible when a time of grieving has resolved the turmoil in our minds?

First, make sure you have as clear a head as you can manage. Keep this in mind when you're tempted to resort to antidepressant or sedative drugs — even if your doctor prescribes them. Sleepless nights won't damage you nearly as much as will too much medication that clouds your reasoning and masks your real grief. Remember Father Hotaling? His warning applies as much to drug-induced peace of mind as to drink.

All of the experts warn about making too many changes, too many life-altering decisions, too quickly. Let the dust settle first — literally. Then look for role models. *I can see you now, saying, This woman has some sort of a fetish about role models.* I'll admit I talk about role models a lot. Because that has worked for me. You might find someone worth emulating in a book about grieving, or a total stranger might appear from out of the blue. No need for you to start at the beginning. ("We met at a pledge dance at Kansas State more than fifty years ago. . . .") Your feelings right now count most. Start with now — but find someone comfortable to talk to.

For example, a new widow whose marriage had seemed perfect came to see me after the death of her husband. I had been single for more than ten years, then. She had no idea of the turmoil caused in my own grieving by drinking. By her standards I had it all together. We talked about loneliness and boredom, a creeping sense of isolation, then she blurted out, "Frankly, I am relieved to be rid of the competition of marriage."

Then she blushed. "Maybe I shouldn't have said that. It sounds so . . . selfish. But it's true. Each decision, big or little, boiled down to who would get his or her own way this time. Ben was a good husband, but that drove me crazy. I don't mean to be disrespectful of the dead, but —"

I looked again at the grieving of other women. Virginia Bigelow read some of her poems to me. Poetry had eased her into acceptance and had started her moving on, and two lines from her scrapbook have stuck with me:

How could you leave me here alone in
    a Noah's Ark world?
At tax time?

Such thoughts ought to be shared. We need to know that those are still *people* we are talking about. Not that we need to pick the old boy to pieces, but we owe it to ourselves to be honest about the past — without

41

letting resentment build up.

Sometimes one remark or question can tell us more than we need to know about a marriage. One recently widowed woman, having a good laugh and a happy time with friends and family, stopped abruptly in her merriment to ask, "Is this all right? Am I too happy too soon?" Hearing just that, everyone who cared about that woman knew her innermost thoughts and could react to her accordingly.

One word of warning: Sometimes a bereaved spouse assumes the role of sole mourner, losing sight of the fact that others — family and friends — feel the loss just as much. Perhaps one of the best perspectives on grieving includes offering consolation to others. Let your kids and grandkids know you share their sorrow. Acknowledge and appreciate their feelings, even in the midst of your own black days.

Grieve? Eventually I did get my new stage of life worked out in my own mind — did move into acceptance and forging ahead. We all work toward this goal of life at our own pace, but we should not avoid the realities by trying to keep life just as it has always been.

Most important, in my fifties I had already initiated some changes in my outlook and active life by beginning a fledgling writing career. This quite naturally involved John. We had a new topic of conversation, an interest new to both of us. Thereby the path had been laid for me with the help and support of my husband before his sudden death. There can be no doubt in my mind that any couple that launch something new and challenging in their lives together — whether as a hobby or as a new life-interest that can be pursued and enjoyed by either of them alone as well as by the two of them together — create a legacy of untold worth when the time comes to face the rest of life alone.

Thank you for allowing me to share the problems that alcohol has caused in my life. Extremely distressing articles appear these days citing the increase in alcoholism among "seniors." We had best stop pontificating about addicted children and start worrying about ourselves. The loss, not only of life-partners but of continued activities, can lead to loneliness and boredom. Booze cannot solve those problems. It can only make them worse.

True confessions time: Writing these chapters has of necessity taken me back through some very hard times. Looking forward beats looking back. Any time.

Chapter Five

Facing Life Alone

Widowhood rearranges the lives of most women. We should expect that, too. Every marriage ends. Some of us fail to realize that fact. Actuarial tables and statistics regularly point out the differences in expected life spans of males and females. Still, occasionally I meet men or women who seem to have been completely surprised by the death of a mate. Some of us apparently consider death to be an option, or a controllable happening.

One of the brighter ladies I know astonished me with her lack of comprehension when her husband died. Finally she sighed and said, "Well, I guess I'll just have to get used to the fact that he isn't here anymore." Tell me, did she have another option? She reminded me of those people who go into sudden anxiety attacks just before Christmas, as if someone had changed the date.

We do have an ostrich-like attitude about death. My husband, a surgeon, talked about dying as a fact of life, which probably accounts for my own pragmatic approach. John used to comment frequently about the family members who refused to face the possibility of death. He pointed out regularly (as if I hadn't paid attention the first time) the words some folks use in avoiding that three-letter word, *die*. "Being gentle or considerate doesn't mean you can't face facts. You didn't 'lose' somebody. You know where they are."

My answer to that comment, which I figured out too late to tell him, makes sense to me: Widowed persons have not "lost" a spouse literally. They simply have not "found" themselves as a single, independent survivor. Their own worth as an individual can come as a complete surprise, particularly after many years of marriage.

With great pleasure I have listened to stories from older women who have discovered they can travel on their own, get the oil changed in the car, meet the insurance payments, find the right man to fix the roof, explore the options of belonging to a different museum, enjoy concerts never appealing to their husbands, or go to the movies by themselves. By the same token, I have loved stories from men who really have fun having their own parties with old friends, scrambling their own eggs, tripping around with one or two grandchildren all to themselves, squiring a variety of widowed friends to all sorts of special events around the old hometown. Granted, widowed men do have the "casserole brigade" to contend with, but most of them seem to consider that a part of the pleasures of old age.

One more thought occurs here — about conversation. None of us looks forward to visiting alone or in a group with some person who tells us incessantly "how George felt about this" or "what John said about that." We must learn to temper our references to our departed spouses and to seek out conversation more suited to the moment. In the company of old friends, even, constant referral to the days gone by amounts to just that: days gone by. After so long a time, it gets old.

But don't impose an inflexible gag rule on yourself. Let your family and friends know when an anniversary, birthday, or graduation brings a flood of feelings and memories to mind. Probably those people you try hardest not to bore with recollections wonder what to say or do, if anything, to make your day easier.

One of the newspaper advice columns carried a letter from a caring son asking what to do about his widowed mother's fiftieth wedding anniversary. Advice: "Say, 'this day will be special to you' to your mother. Take her out or give her a small gift."

That column encouraged me to mention my own forty-fifth wedding anniversary to two teenagers — a granddaughter and a niece — while they visited me in Lake George, New York. Those two kids acted as if they had not heard me. Then on a Sunday morning as I returned from church (half mad because they had "slept in"), I found a note: "Oma, change your clothes and come to the dock."

At the dock I found two busy, happy girls who had festooned my little inflatable boat with bright towels, prepared an impressive lunch from my refrigerator, and made greeting cards and garlands. They escorted me on a floating picnic as if the Queen Mother had arrived.

I could have kept still and pouted most of the day about that uncelebrated anniversary, but I'm glad I chose not to.

Getting older means good times ahead when we accept the reality of this stage of our lives.

Chapter Six

Grief — Write It Out!

It happens in our lives more often than some of us realize: The solution to a puzzling problem comes from someone totally unaware of our dilemma. Like in the supermarket this morning. A most pleasant-looking woman stopped near the check-out stands to say hello. She complimented me on my little travel "fillers" on TV, which I surely appreciated, but then she said something more.

"I really enjoy the way you write. My husband used to say, 'Now, you could write like Frances,' and he bought me a word processor before he died. So I'm writing and loving it."

Here I had been pondering whether or not I should include the therapy of writing in terms of coping with grief. Did that belong in this book, or had I been unique in finally turning to writing? Would readers relate?

Mrs. Peterson had answered that question. With or without a word processor, writing about the losses and the changes in our lives can make a difference.

The Widow's Handbook by Charlotte-Barron and Carol Cozart had caught my attention with the suggestion, "Try writing a letter to your late husband. . . ." That worked wonders for me, but apparently not until I had reached a certain point. I had to approach this letter-writing cautiously, for reasons I'll never understand. First I wrote a memorial essay about my mother-in-law, Vesta. That paved the way for the "confrontation" of a letter to John.

VESTA

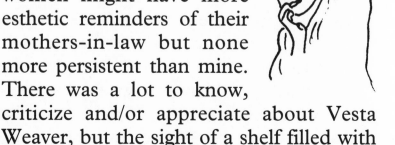

Whenever I buy White Cloud bathroom tissue I think of Vesta. Other women might have more esthetic reminders of their mothers-in-law but none more persistent than mine. There was a lot to know, criticize and/or appreciate about Vesta Weaver, but the sight of a shelf filled with toilet paper distills for me the woman, her character and her life. Especially the end of her life.

In July, 1965, Vesta and I went to the grocery store together for the last time. Her husband, Joe, went with us for a change. Before leaving the house Vesta prepared a list written with obvious care and effort. As I drove down Republican Street to downtown Concordia, Kansas, on that hot day, Vesta was explaining the grocery list and the process of shopping to Joe as she would to a small child with a handful of dimes.

When I parked the car in the lot next to Bogart's Market, I swallowed hard. This would not be easy. Joe Weaver was seventy years old. Until this summer he had never shopped for groceries, not in his whole life. That was Vesta's job.

"You're going to need to know how to do this, Joe," she said quietly as we got out of the car. "It can be fun. Relax."

Inside the store she pointed out the aisles of cereal, dog food, cleaning supplies and paper products. Joe walked ahead of us with the cart.

"This is the third time we've done this," she whispered to me. "Watch. He misses about half the list but he always buys toilet paper."

"Toilet paper?"

"That's it. Every time he buys more toilet paper. We must have a six-month supply from the last two trips. There he goes again."

Vesta's cotton house dress hung from her once-broad shoulders like a shroud. Her eyes shone in her bony face. Even her eyeglasses and false teeth seemed too big. She took my arm for support, then smiled.

Joe and I carried the sacks to the kitchen table. Vesta insisted that he put all the supplies away himself. "You'll need to know where things are."

Knowing where anything was had always been Vesta's job.

Vesta and I talked a lot during that visit, just as we had through the twenty years we had been in-laws. She was the most pragmatic woman I shall ever know. She made a fetish of being down-to-earth, unspoiled. Having *no* affectations was almost an affectation.

"Cheese is cheese," she'd remark when I would proudly present a gourmet recipe. "No sense in all those fancy foreign names. We'll use good old rat-trap cheese."

When the bed was unmade: "It felt good

51

when you got out of it this morning, didn't it?"

She was Vesta to everyone in town, even her children and grandchildren. "None of that high-sounding Mrs. Weaver stuff for me or some cutesy name like Mumsie or Granny. Just call me Vesta. That's my name."

Grandkids loved to visit. Rides in the country with Joe and Vesta were childhood treats, especially when Vesta would whistle or hum. Her voice was a little like a calliope but a ride over to the old family farm was reason for rejoicing, so Vesta sang. When Joe's driving was too much "like Barney Oldfield," Vesta changed her tune to "Nearer My God to Thee." The children squealed and Joe slowed down.

About a spot on a skirt or a child's uncombed hair Vesta would say, "A man on a galloping horse would never see it."

About cancer when the surgeons simply closed her abdomen — no hope of recovery: "They say one person in four is going to die of cancer. I don't know why I wouldn't be one of them."

Facing reality, even terminal cancer, was not anything her husband was ready to do. That was Vesta's job, too: facing reality. The arrangement they called marriage was a simple one. Joe worked at the post office. Vesta worked at everything else.

Growing up on a farm in Cloud County, Kansas, had not been a childhood filled with wonder and delight. Motherless at seven or eight, Vesta had cared for her brother and sister and had taken orders from her father. After two years of college ("enough for any girl . . ."), she married and took orders from Joe. To her that was the way life goes.

Never in her life did she wear high heels or slacks or a diamond ring. Never did she play bridge or go to lunch with the girls. Never did she go the forty miles to Salina to shop. She never had a car or a bank account of her own. Neither in her own mind did she lack the absolute necessities of life. I never heard her whine. Never saw her complain.

In the summer of her forty-eighth year of marriage she said, "I guess I should have seen to it Joe could take care of himself. It's hard for him to learn now." My insides churned and my face must have been crimson recalling the hundreds — thousands — of times I had sworn under my breath at that chauvinistic sonovabitch demanding to be waited on with the same smug, "That's Vesta's job."

In those last months she showed him how to wash his clothes, do his dishes, iron shirts, pay utility bills, find socks, get the car serviced, mow the lawn, and call the plumber. She taught him about frozen foods and about how to operate the can opener. She demonstrated changing sheets when she could scarcely stand.

Then in August of 1965, satisfied that she had done the best she could to prepare her husband for life without her, she took to her bed and died as matter-of-factly as she had lived. "Don't take me back to the hospital," she commanded. "I'll have to be here to make sure Joe gets along all right." She helped him find her good black dress, arranged for her sister to braid her hair.

So the priest came and she said her prayers and that was that.

Vesta Weaver had never considered herself "special." I don't think she had any idea of how much she was respected for her let's-just-get-on-with-it attitude. She would have been astonished by her own funeral. The church and the parish hall were filled to overflowing with her friends and admirers. The bishop came from Topeka. Senator Carlson came from Washington. Vesta had made her point:

That's the way life is.

She was quite a woman. I never really understood the way she lived, but I certainly learned a lot from the way she died.

That memorial for Vesta prompted thoughts of writing something special about John. By this time I no longer regarded myself a grieving widow. Instead, I had developed a growing pride in the way my life had progressed. I found myself wishing to share those thoughts with him.

Our courtship had consisted mainly of letters during the war. Why not write letters now? I include just one. Others written later tended to repeat a lot of what I've said here. No wonder he often remarked, "It's not what you say, Frances, it's how often you say it!"

Dear John,
The Bears are beating the Vikings. That same old Sunday afternoon sound brings you right up front here. I am now sitting in the Atlanta airport, corner table in a crowded bar. I cannot even see the screen of the TV but the sound suffices. Sunday afternoon football. This provides an appropriate backdrop for commencing a series of letters to you even though you have

not watched nor slept through the past ten NFL seasons. I'll not see (hear) all of this game because I have a plane to catch. Next stop, La Guardia; then Princeton, Detroit, Saratoga Springs, Rome (New York), and Portland, Oregon, before I get back to Pueblo in a couple of weeks. I'll explain all of this travel later. Right now I'm caught up in this football crowd.

(Surely you have not forgotten sleeping in front of TV, especially football. Remember the Monday night when I suggested, "Why don't you just go to bed if you're so tired?"

You said, "What time is it?"

I said, "Nine o'clock."

You said, "Too early for bed. Wake me at nine-thirty.")

Men's voices, men's laughter, men's shop talk about cars, small talk about big deals — all this talk drifts over to the corner — but football sounds rule the day. Sunday sounds of you and me and the Broncos and the Raiders and the Redskins and the Rams. So I choose this place to reminisce, writing a letter to you.

I guess I write a letter to you like this every ten years whether I need to or not. (I can hear you saying, "That's what the girls in Concordia used to say.") More precisely, ten years, nine months and three weeks. I figure this catch-up will be a lengthy process since I have so much to say but I am aiming to have this letter finished for you on our eleventh anniversary. That makes the deadline January 10, 1991, doesn't it? Our eleventh anniversary. Mine of being single, yours of being dead.

Saying "dead" stops most people in their tracks, you know, John. You used to complain about that a lot — the patients who could not bring themselves to face the facts of living and dying, so they couldn't say "dead" right out loud. They used some euphemism like "passed away." You had a tendency to be pretty judgmental about that. How you would have loved a lady I met in Portland, Oregon, who claimed the oft-used statement, "I lost my husband," sounds careless. Like, "I can't find my eyeglasses." You did dislike my habit of saying "you know" all the time, too, John. Did you notice it in the first of this paragraph? Sorry.

In some ways death might have separated us just yesterday. Other ways, it seems ages since we were at home in Beulah and you went up to bed before I did on that Thursday night. An hour later, you didn't reach to turn off the light over your side of the bed when I came up. Then I knew.

John, do you remember how we laughed and made fun of those endless Christmas letters and poems we used to get about the wonders of everyone else's families? Patty bragged about kids who blew horns and shot baskets while she "baked the best homemade bread on the block." Aunt Grace tried to tell us all about Evelyn's twenty-one living children and their families, all on the back of one Hallmark card. This letter will be a lot like that.

Rolling more than a decade into one series of letters could be a real bore. I'll skip some details, and I'll put in a few laughs as we go along. Whenever the kids and I start reminiscing we always wind up laughing. I like to think that speaks well for our family. I also might strike a nerve or two to make you mad. Most of all, I want you to know how much a part of our lives you are now. The melody lingers on, as the girls back in Concordia used to say.

(Incidentally, did I ever make it clear to you how sick I got of hearing about the girls in Concordia? Are all men that way about hometown sweethearts, or were those girls special?)

Catching up on how much and how fast the world has changed in the past eleven years would be a hopeless task. *Fax* and *Sprint* you can get along without knowing. I do harbor a vague feeling that you know a lot about what goes on around here. Your powers of observation always astounded me, particularly when I thought I'd gotten away with something. You saw. You knew. That has to be what made you such an extraordinary diagnostician. And I feel timid, like a little kid afraid of being scolded, as I write this now.

You managed to take a history and physical of everyone we met, patient or not. I picked up much of that from you and it comes in handy in this new part of my life. Thank you.

As a matter of strict fact, I can thank you for enhancing much of what my life has become since your sudden departure. Also, I find myself feeling cheated, or at least short-changed, by some of our married-life experiences. Looking at the grandkids, I regret the good times you have missed, but we cannot do much about that. That's what these letters are all about, John. After all these years I feel the need, the readiness, to go over it with you. Don't worry, I won't cause as much trauma as our monthly bouts with the checkbook. You might even enjoy this process. So relax, dear John, but keep your feet braced.

Some of the women you and I have known for years are moping around, claiming to be the only women in the world whose husbands have died and left them here. Some are even mad about it. Frankly, I think "here" is a pretty good place to be, and I am more than certain you would have felt the same way had you been the one to be "remaindered." I just made up this term for this condition of widowhood. Rather calls to mind the tables of cut-rate books in B. Dalton or Waldenbooks, the books nobody would buy at full price. A real bargain for some lucky soul, huh?

I am also certain you would not have remained on the bargain table for very long. You might have had a hard time deciding between the two obvious candidates for Mrs. Weaverhood, but like most men, you would not have been single for long. Statistics prove that. Far more older women than men live alone. I almost added, "You know."

Let's get back for one moment to the subject of pre-planning funeral services and such. You were most specific, probably because you had heard so much about the subject from your father. You were not as monotonous as Joe, thank heavens. As a matter of fact, you detested Joe's incessant trips to the cemetery to visit Vesta's grave because he could have put some of that thoughtfulness into caring for her while she was alive. Agreed. But you were almost comically insistent about wanting to be cremated and buried in the Beulah Cemetery. Everyone laughed when you explained your reasoning: the Beulah lots were cheap, and the view was spectacular. You did want the ashes buried and a permanent marker. Good for you, John. None of us sat around wondering or whispering about what Old Dad would want us to do. You made that clear. I've followed your example and have the whole thing on file at Ascension Church, but I've included a postlude of "Onward Christian Soldiers" at top volume. We should have thrown that in for you. We did have your ashes moved into Pueblo after Ascension built the columbarium, but we left the marker in Beulah. Since you always wanted an epitaph, I put on the stone the best for you I could come up with, simply: "He gave . . ." Anyone seeing the stone can finish the sentence according to their experience of knowing you. I'm proud of that. I put on all the initials after your name. Important, to say the least.

So there's another plus for our ledger. You made those decisions and those days easier for all of us. Thanks.

When you hear "Onward Christian Soldiers" rattling the north end of Pueblo, you'll know I'm on my way.

Love
Fran

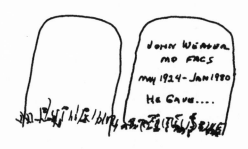

Chapter Seven

Downhill Slide

Most of my life needed attention in my early fifties. Much as I scorned any discussion of the "empty-nest syndrome," I fell victim to it without realizing it. "Frantic" could have described that time, as one project after another occurred, only to be dropped or ignored.

Only in the past year since my daughter, Allison, has reached this stage of her life have I fully recognized the pace I set for myself in near-desperate attempts to convince the world and myself how very valuable I was. For instance, Allison has been on a redecorating/paint-the-walls spree and has taken on bigger and bigger jobs with the historical society in her town. When I was her age (fifty) I made all new chair seats for eight dining room chairs — crewel work, yet — with elaborate patterns. To force myself to finish this enormous (for me) project, I replaced each seat as I finished the new one. That way the chairs no longer matched until the last seat cover made it to the eighth chair. This took months, of course, and visitors devastated me when they failed to rave over this great achievement. Resentment and frustration took over.

Reestablishing a sense of accomplishment stretched farther and farther, reaching new heights when I bought a second-hand Hammond organ, probably cast off from a funeral parlor, in order to play piano–organ duets. A dear friend of long standing from down the road agreed to be roped into this — she must have sensed my frustration since she's a much more accomplished musician than I — and we spent hours filling the air and the ears of anyone unlucky enough to be in the neighborhood with renditions of "Whispering" and "Don't Blame Me." Neva Jo sounded great on the piano. I stumbled along on the organ. But it gave us something to do for a while.

As with many of the women I knew, entertaining reached new highs (or new lows) at the same time. Any season or holiday called for a party. What else should we do? With the kids out on their own (at least for a while), our husbands busy, combined with the sameness of being perennial chairmen of every fund drive, we threw ourselves into having a good time.

My most-special attraction I called "Clean the Creek Week." Our house sat beside a mountain stream. Fall and winter left dead branches and other rubbish along the banks. What should have taken me one hour of concerted cleanup turned into hours of preparation of "fabulous" picnic food and clever invitations, plus unlimited bloody Marys or screwdrivers. Thirty or forty women drove thirty miles out to our mountain home for the festivities. Some fell in the creek. All claimed to have had a glorious time swinging rakes, shovels, and clippers. They had to listen to a piano–organ recital and then they headed for home. John actually cleaned the creek on the Saturday morning of his next weekend off.

What I am saying here boils down to a frightening (in retrospect) emotional instability: I was looking for one more useful project, one more way to convince myself and the world that I was not to be discarded because my principal job (mothering) seemed to have come to an end. Reality — or glimpses thereof — led to talking with a psychiatrist. After several sessions of hearing myself repeating the same complaints and the same defects in my life, that line of attack seemed fruitless. Besides, all of those accounts of my worries and shortcomings turned out to be someone else's fault when I told the story.

The doctor did make me take a long look at the earlier years of matronhood. That way I made more sense of the lifestyle that had me stymied when the time arrived to face this age-old middle-age change of life. (Our mothers had the right spin on that one!) In every neighborhood I knew back in the fifties, all mothers operated in direct competition with Donna Reed and June Cleaver. The perfect image of Mom fixing a good hot breakfast — two well-scrubbed kids who found their own socks and ate their oatmeal without a whimper — tarnished forever the mother image in our house.

Our families watched TV families whose greatest trauma involved someone being left out of the neighbor's birthday party. I had aspired to be favorably compared to Donna Reed for more than thirty years and never made the grade. (*Note.* This just occurred to me: Our teenage sons' favorite TV show, "Bonanza," had no mother!)

At that time, when I most needed help without knowing what had happened, Peggy

Gandy came along. Now, I know I would have caught on to the advantages of this next

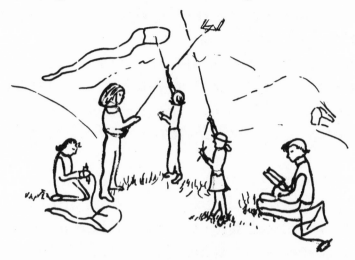

stage of my life sooner or later. But a role model always helps. Peggy served as a catalyst. She convinced six of us to fly kites — without our children. During the past twenty years, I have told and retold the tale of our kite-flying group. Suffice it to say here, flying those kites, insignificant as that seemed, triggered for us the understanding of our lives. We learned (because of the unstructured activity and the freedom of spirit felt as those kites soared above our mountain meadows) that our lives could expand in the same way those kites would catch a breeze and go!

Here is a little something I keep on my refrigerator. It serves as a memorial to my remarkable friend Peggy, who led me to fly kites and to other freedoms:

The most visible creators I know of are those artists whose medium is life itself, the ones who express the impossible — without brush, hammer, clay or guitar. They neither paint nor sculpt — their medium is being. *Whatever their presence touches has increased life. They see and don't have to draw. They are the artists of being alive.*

I have no idea who wrote those words, but they describe precisely my own impression of this woman who had been diagnosed with cancer early on when her second child was born. Peggy lived by that diagnosis, fully aware that "her days were numbered" because of the type of disease she had. Every day meant something special: another chance to experience more of life and share it. Although she never mentioned this to her friends, in the last days of her life we all knew. She enhanced the lives of many folks including the Beulah Valley Association for Tethered Flight. Whatever came along, Peggy made the most of it.

On a plane I talked with a truly distinguished-looking woman obviously headed for a most important meeting of some sort. She ruffled through files of official-looking papers, sorting and considering each one.

Finally she apologized for such a disturbance, but remarked about the necessity to know exactly the facts of the upcoming meeting in Pasadena. Positive she had a position on the national board of some corporation, I asked about the nature of her trip.

"Rabbit breeders. I'm going to a meeting of rabbit breeders. As a matter of fact, I have eighteen of my own rabbits with me."

In her ensuing explanation, I learned that rabbits had done for her what kites and Peggy had done for me. "I just sat around wondering what to do after the children left home and my husband died. I thought about rabbits. Why not? I had always been fascinated by rabbits but never owned one. So I became a breeder and this has opened an entire new world for me. I'm busier than ever."

I heard the same sort of story from a woman in Connecticut, a single woman who appeared on a talk show to discuss a craft fair of great magnitude. I asked about her talent and interest in crafts of all sorts. She, too, could have been talking about kites: "I chose to stay at home with my mother when she had Alzheimer's. She just sat in front of the TV all day but I stayed with her. She didn't know I was there. But *I* knew, even though the boredom, day after day, really got to me. One day I picked up some of the embroidery stuff Mother used to use and made a bib out of a washcloth. I could sit with her and do that, at least. Eventually I became so hooked on all the possibilities of making things that I had given everyone in the neighborhood all sorts of stuff, and they raved about my work.

"After my mother died I thought I could go back to my old job. They said I was too old. I felt terrible for a while, then went to a craft fair. The next week I made all sorts of things to take to the next craft fair and I've been busier and happier than ever before. A whole new world exists in craft fairs all over the country. I have new friends. I have an entirely unexpected new interest in life."

The operative word in that last sentence is *unexpected.* At least, that applies to my own life. If someone had told me fifteen years ago I'd sit here at a word processor recounting my own rite of passage into these penultimate years, I'd have laughed in his — or her — face. No way would I become a writer. But kites made it happen. Kites and being in the right place and the right frame of mind at the right time.

I like that word, *penultimate.* The *Oxford Dictionary* defines it as "last but one." If it didn't sound so stuffy, I'd use it more to define this stage of our lives. This can also be termed a "time of final options." If we find a way to add interest and importance (for ourselves) to these later years, we have accomplished a lot for our family as well as for ourselves.

Kite-flying led me to writing, which had never entered my mind as a serious consideration of something I might do. But Peggy and the kites had opened new doors. When the suggestion came that we should share the joy of kiting through writing to a column called "Off Hours" in the *National Observer*, extolling the wonders of a twenty-five-foot Mylar dragon on the back of a rolling wind, I jumped at the chance to express my own pleasure in this unexpected way.

With the acceptance of my dissertation on kite-flying for older folks, and the subsequent failure to see it in print (because the newspaper folded), I felt a new sensation. Exhilaration and disappointment combined to propel me into action when a newspaper editor in New York suggested submission of my meager effort to magazines. Talk about new worlds! Learning about magazine submission and acceptance and publication opened my head as it had not been working in a long time. Eventual acceptance of the article and payment (!) by *Vogue* came as a complete surprise. Not a surprise about magazines or writers, but about myself.

Happily, this revelation of unused skills of my own not only affected me, it delighted John. When some of the whiners I meet say, "Oh, but you found a new lease on life because you're a widow," I can tell them truthfully that a small change in my own outlook brought about a welcome change in our marriage. Single women aren't the only ones who can discover unknown talents and make changes in their lives. Anyone, at any age, can surprise himself or herself. The joy of discovery tends to become contagious.

My newfound interest in kites pleased him. John liked kites. We flew them on our own, away from my group. He also took an active interest in the writing. Our conversations took a giant step from "What went wrong today?" to "What did you see worth writing about today?"

We had a new view of our old world. Subjects for articles discussed during moments together often spurred weekend trips. We explored and expanded upon many shared interests and uncovered new ways of considering old topics. In short, we became more interesting to each other, to our old friends, and to our family. On Sunday afternoons when the kids came out to see us, lively conversations about reading and writing dominated the talk around the dinner table. I had met new people when I had ventured to travel on my own to a couple of writers' workshops. This pleased all of us.

Thus it happened that John's death — suddenly — came when he had actually helped me to lay the groundwork for my life in these senior years, with or without him. The new evaluation of my own capabilities and my own worth did not make the shock of his dying any less, but it did make coping with the reality of life on my own much more palatable.

One of the fine women who have been role models for me, Skippy Salfeety, told me, "We all must have three things: someone to love, something to do, and something to look forward to." Well, in my family I had plenty of someones to love, and with the writing I would have plenty to do, and much more than I ever dreamed of to look forward to.

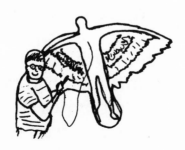

Chapter Eight

A Little Learning Goes a Long Way

When I began to write I began to think. In some wondrous unexpected way a perhaps dormant part of my brain took fire, spewing out words and phrases and, most especially, thoughts that surprised and delighted me. Had I been Dumb Dora for all of those years of matronhood?

Speaking of which, isn't that a good word, *matronhood?* I did not make it up. The *Concise Oxford Dictionary* defines *matron* as "a woman managing domestic arrangements, hence matronship, matronage, and matronhood." The use of that word on this page demonstrates precisely what I want to say here.

When I began to write I began to think in very different terms than had been my habit for a long time. Old phrases and comfortable expressions had to give way to new, inventive ideas and concise sentences. Writing challenged any skills I could dig up from school days and nurtured new ways of evaluating my own thought processes. One basic became clear: I wrote not to change the world but to change myself. This new view of my world excited me more than had anything since I suddenly understood my chemistry professor back at Kansas State. No wonder John approved. Any change stimulates, and this one certainly did that.

Following that first magazine article, I found writers' workshops and seminars. Taking notes, just handling a yellow tablet and pen and paying attention for my own edification, gave me a charge not felt in years. Before widowhood, while participating in a writers' weekend, I had become aware of older students having a great time at Adirondack Community College, studying what they really wanted to know. Little did I dream it would soon be my turn.

During those matronage decades, the Wednesday Morning Club and my P.E.O. chapter meetings had filled some of the need for mental stimulation. I appreciated that. The ladies of "the club" (the oldest study club for women in Colorado) had a history of each member presenting one book review or research paper during the year. Some very smart ladies gave wonderful programs. I never left a meeting without feeling I had learned something. Same with the sisterhood of P.E.O., which is based on a thirst for knowledge and scholarship more than a hundred years old.

These at least made me think once or twice a week. During my active political days I studied up on the issues and some of the history involved. I prided myself on my ability to come up with the right answers when the youngsters needed help with homework. In other words, I used but did not stretch my brain. Not learning much new, just making use of stored material, you might say.

Going back to the college classroom opened so many doors I astonished myself and my family. Professor Jean Rikhoff, herself a fine writer, conducted her creative-writing class in a way that was totally new to me. Each student brought enough copies of the assigned work for all members of the group. I could not even type. (I still can't!) To write an acceptable piece for the class was a joy. To make one readable copy to be recopied for class distribution almost drove me crazy. I'd get to the middle of a page and discover nineteen typos and start over. I considered buying that white-out goop by the gallon. The frustration of such a problem in the early eighties challenged this return student more than I had anticipated.

As has happened often in these blooming years of mine (more about that later), the gods of creativity and mental restoration rode with me on the plane when I went home to Colorado for Christmas that first semester. A bright, talkative young man seated next to me listened patiently as I recounted the pitfalls of going to college to learn to write when I couldn't even type.

Wonder of wonders, this guy sold word processors for Olympia. I had barely heard of word processing in 1982. Nobody I knew used one of those gadgets. This young man made a lot of sense, convinced me to try it out, and gave me his card. During my vacation from school, I read Peter McWilliams' book about word processors, and devoured every word. The first thing I did when I got back to my off-season motel room at Lake George, New York, was call that man about an Olympia.

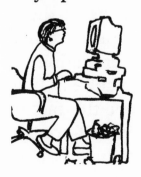 My life changed again, literally. That original 1980s machine consisted of a big electronic typewriter that served as keyboard and printer, and a computer

screen where I could see and correct my mistakes before making class copies of my assignments. The machine also turned out as many copies as needed. Miraculous! Since that point I have steadily upgraded my equipment, but WordStar will always stand by me until I master typing.

The learning process continues. Once in a while I am reminded of those doldrum days when I nearly gave in to the stereotypical symptoms of over-the-hill life. But then I am constantly reminded of the vast difference in my own life that resulted from continuing education.

One of the greatest advances in old-age-coping in recent years has taken place on college campuses, in museums, and in learning-oriented tour groups around the world. The emphasis on continuing education makes a bigger difference in our aging lives than any other single phenomenon. I realize that, more than any other aspect of older years, the opportunity for lifelong learning has made the biggest difference in the lives my sisters and I have compared with our own grandmother and her generation.

We all need to know ourselves. I knew myself well enough to accept the fact that, now that I had regained my self-control in the social world, I would not make the most of a college career by staying at home in Colorado and enrolling at the local schools. The problem lay with me, not the schools. As sure as anything, I'd start some class with great enthusiasm, only to be interrupted in my studies by the phone. "Can you be the chairman? You have lots of time, now." Or "Gertrude has a cold. Can you fill in for bridge today? You can do that homework later. *We* need you. We're your *friends*."

What I had to do was paint myself into a corner. Simply, to go far enough away that I separated myself from daily temptations to take the easy way, lunch at the club, hang out with the kids. Where would that lead me in this last 20 percent of my life? Nowhere. If I had stayed at home as widows have generally done, waiting for the family to call, playing bridge with the same bunch, going to the same cocktail parties, having the same conversations I had enjoyed for the past thirty years, I would have missed the greatest time of personal growth I have ever imagined possible for an older woman. All because I discovered I could still learn, and that I loved learning more than ever.

Adirondack Community College typifies the college most accessible to returning students of any age. The campus, on the edge of Glens Falls, New York, consists of half a dozen new buildings — no ivy-covered halls here. With the advice of My Friend the Professor (Jean Rikhoff), I enrolled in creative writing, cultural anthropology, Spanish, basic design, and poetry. Since ACC has no dorms, I lived in a motel at nearby Lake George, the Queen of American Lakes and one of the most important sites in early-American history.

My life was enchanted, a schoolgirl all the way. In this town I had no history. Never had I chaired a committee; nobody claimed me as a sister, mother, daughter, wife. My friends, most of them single, had college connections or wrote for a living. These people became my support group, though I did not tell them so. That change in social contacts almost outweighed the classes in learning new living skills and adopting a changed set of values. For a traditional housewife of thirty-four years, that step alone was like taking three giant steps without saying, "Mother, may I?"

Returning students play an important role in today's colleges and universities. They display an enthusiasm and dedication about learning whatever comes along. The class discussions take on a wider dimension with older students drawing on personal experience.

For example, in cultural anthropology the chapters and class sessions took on added interest and importance when we studied the Zuñi, whom I had visited. The Zuñi culture does not recognize ownership of personal property. Whatever they have can be used by whoever needs it at the moment. So say the anthropologists.

That explained to me why, when John and I had visited the Zuñi pueblo, looking around the fancy "native crafts shop" built by some government agency, we found Anglo people manning the store.

"I thought this would be for the Zuñi. Run by their own people," John had remarked to the officious clerk.

"We started out that way, but those Native Americans stole each other blind from the first day, so we had to take over. They couldn't make money in an operation like that."

There in the classroom, reading that textbook of cultural anthropology, I understood at last why those Zuñi behaved as they had in that shop. Why hadn't those do-good professionals known about the Zuñi belief in communal property?

If every day I learn this much about the world I think I know, I'll wind up smarter about all sorts of things, I thought. I also decided that anthropology should be a basic required course for all students in any school.

Other older folks in the class had more to add to the textbook. The youngsters apparently had an added interest because we old folks "knew so much." And I learned new words such as *ethnocentricity* and *atavism* that come to mind with every new headline about territorial disputes around today's world.

During that two years of college life I grew as much as I had during my first college career, maybe more. I surely learned more about life in general and writing in particular. One week, a fellow student and I took off for Washington, DC, for a Smithsonian seminar on magazine writing. The instructor, Edwards Park, wrote the column "Around the Mall and Beyond" in the *Smithsonian* magazine. I admired his work. This chance could not be missed.

One concentrated week of classes and homework — writing short nonfiction — convinced me that column-writing offered the best opportunity for someone like me. I had no aspirations of becoming a famous writer or the author of the great American novel. Instead, writing opened for me new doors of awareness and opportunity, a different way to look at the world 400 words at a crack. Mr. Park also stressed using fiction techniques for nonfiction — that is, adding dialogue and that sort of thing to a narrative piece. Invaluable to me over ten years of columns.

Here's one example: Mr. Park sent us into the Smithsonian museum rooms. The men went to the display of First Ladies' gowns. The women in the class studied the "John Bull," a steam locomotive from the nineteenth century. Our assignment was to describe what we saw. "Experience writing about something you *don't* know about — men with dresses, women with locomotives," he said. "Make it interesting on your own terms."

Recalling lessons about word association and right-brain creativity from Gabriele Rico's wonderful book, *Writing the Natural Way*, I studied "John Bull" from top to bottom, trying to notice details. Then, using Rico's "clustering" method of thought and word progression, I came up with this story. Without her "Natural Way," I certainly would have written a much more factual, less interesting, piece.

JERKWATER, NEW JERSEY
Fran Weaver

First we heard it — then we felt it —
then we saw it. We kids would race
down through the trees behind the
school to watch the men put the water
in to make the steam to run the train.
It always made me mad that the boys
got there first. My dumb old skirts
caught on the brambles so I couldn't
run, but I got to the tracks before the
other girls, anyway. Every Tuesday and
Thursday about 3:45 — in the fall of
forty-three.

The whistle made a wheeping sound
like nothing else in the world — "wheep,
wheep, wheep" — three times. That was
the signal for the man at the tracks to
be ready. Then, even before we could
see it coming through the trees around
the curve, we felt it. The ground started

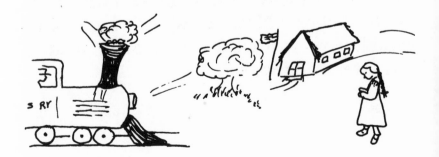

to shake — an excitement coming through our feet. The littlest kids wanted to touch the rails, but the man wouldn't let them. We almost wet our pants jumping up and down, waiting.

Louder and louder the sounds of the train were — almost to make us deaf — the puffing steam, the rattling boxes of freight, the heavy barrels bouncing around — and the wheels clacking on the tracks closer and closer to us. By the time we could see him, "John Bull," we couldn't hear each other talk.

What a sight that was; the wondrous black engine spouting steam, the shiny copper pipes and valves — the brass bell clanging, clanging — and the great black cowcatcher out in front.

Then came the smoke and the ashes. Some days the cinders and soot were just all over the place. We ran across the tracks when the wind was blowing at us so we wouldn't get covered with 'em. My eyes would get full of thick smoke that hurt nearly to make me cry and the stinging inside my nose went clear down in my chest. The black stuff that landed on my clothes made big smears when I tried to brush it off. That made Mamma really mad and she'd say we must come right home and not even wait to see "John Bull."

Finally the brakeman on the open car stood with his feet wide apart and pulled with all his might on the big handle. The screeching of the stopping wheels was the loudest noise of all. Then it was quiet except for a little puffing, and the train men waved to us kids as we headed on home from school.

Mr. Park and the class approved, and I was tickled silly about the different way I had found to create interest in my own writing. I felt I had described the train so that my readers actually saw it.

Many older people have a variety of reasons for returning to school. For each one, today's world holds the answer, the ways and means. I have spent lots of time with Elderhostel. One week at a time, learning in the company of other oldsters not talking about their bad backs, weak bladders, and rotten sons-in-law not only informs but renews our confidence in the older world.

Writers' groups have contributed almost as much as college to the regeneration of Frances Weaver. Once again, this support for a fledgling writer intent on improving her life and herself proved invaluable.

The International Women's Writing Guild, with the remarkable leadership of Hannelore Hahn, set me on my way to the writing world. Beginning with the astonishing position of being "kite-flier in residence" at an IWWG conference at Skidmore College in Saratoga Springs, New York, I continued as a participant and board member for years, by which I profited immensely. As a matter of strict fact, that introduction to upstate New York sold me on that marvelous part of our country, so when it came time to go to college again and to have a second home, I stuck to that area. At the same time, the Santa Barbara Writers Conference continues to be not only most congenial but a reason to do better.

During these years of college-appreciation and additional learning opportunities, I have self-published eight books, written ten years' worth of columns, been featured in a PBS "filler" that has been shown around the country, plus had many other wondrous, undreamed-of experiences, which I'll recount elsewhere — and all because I went back to college. Without that move, none of this (get that: *none of this*) would have happened. (So far, I'm not making a lot of money. But the profits are enormous!)

Knowing the impact of continuing education in my own life, I have used whatever I can afford along the way to establish a scholarship for older women at my alma mater, Kansas State University. A bequest from a cousin beefed up the scholarship considerably, so now it is functioning. Understanding the importance of keeping our minds alert and alive, acquiring new skills, and exploring new worlds certainly did not enter into my grandmother's life, but it does mine. And it might in yours, too!

As a matter of fact, the more I consider and discuss continuing education the more I discover the opportunities. In your own hometown you can probably find any number of classes and courses offered for older students. The community college here in Pueblo has developed an outstanding curriculum for oldsters that can be fitted into our workaday world. I'll bet a call to your local community college would surprise you if you haven't already found out what's available.

I've mentioned the writing seminar at the Smithsonian. For years I have maintained a contributing membership in that venerable institution in order to receive the magazine and stay informed about the myriad seminars and tours conducted under the auspices of the Smithsonian. After all, it belongs to all of us. In groups accompanied by experts in art history, geology, world history, and anthropology, I have studied in Colorado Indian ruins, Puget Sound, Tuscany, France, and Italy — many places with wonder and satisfaction.

The back pages of the *Smithsonian* magazine, "The Smithsonian Traveler," list excursions for learning, any one of which appeals to me. For example: "Kenya Safari for Families," "Yucatan Adventure," "Big Cats of Tanzania," "Red Sea Passage," "Insights into India's Heritage," "Wildlife of Costa Rica," "Treasures of Ancient Egypt."

But that's only a part of the first column. How about "U.S. and Canada Tours: Toronto and Beyond," "New York Landmarks," "Christmas in Savannah," "Baja Whale Watch," "Canyons and Cultures of the Southwest," "Birding in South Texas"? Or how about seminars the likes of "Cuisines of Philadelphia," "Rock Art of the Southwest," "Baseball (at Cooperstown, New York)," "Polar Bears," "American Antique Furniture," "Coral Reef Ecology"?

Also on this incredible list we can find Odyssey Tours titled "France through the Ages," "Legacy of the Inca," or "Moscow and St. Petersburg."

That's enough from me to let you know

how much we can learn in exceedingly pleasant surroundings. You can get a free catalog with 300 listings by calling or writing the Smithsonian, MRC 702, Washington DC 20560.

Honestly, I do not work for the Smithsonian or for Elderhostel, but they work for me. If you have somehow missed finding out about Elderhostel, I surely cannot tell the whole story. It's bigger than both of us. Don't just sit there! Send a postcard to Elderhostel, Inc., 75 Federal Street, Boston, MA 02110-1941. Those good people will send you all you ever wanted to know about this continuing education worldwide.

What? Where? How about Jekyll Island, Georgia, for a week studying Chaucer, Lord Byron, or Tennessee Williams, plus the Big Band era and the American Family? Or a week in California where one Elderhostel in a garden resort at Palm Desert offers a history of the desert, history of dates and citrus, and golf for everyone!

In the Poconos of Pennsylvania you can practice nature photography and start your own family history in the same week. International Elderhostel takes us as far afield as Beijing and Bali, Scandinavia and South Africa.

Try it. You'll like it.

Chapter Nine

What Shall I Do Now?

Catfish nuggets, fried green tomatoes, corn on the cob, tossed green salad, fresh peaches, and cookies. I had that for supper the other night. Cooked it myself. What restaurant in your town has such a menu, plus friendly service, soft lights, a quiet place to carry on a conversation, and no tipping? If such a place exists in our town I don't know about it. What better reason for spending "quality time" with friends in our own homes?

You have probably seen, as I have, lines of older folks forming outside restaurants (especially in Florida) for the "early bird" dinners. Some of these crowds gather before 5:00, waiting. They eat early because their crowd does, then they get back home and wait for dark so they can go to bed. Whenever I see these people — bored, grim-faced, determined to hold their place in the line against all comers — I recall a marvelous conversation with some of the club women I met at Beverly Hills, Florida, several years ago.

In a planning session for a club luncheon, conversation turned to "Since we moved down from Iowa, I haven't even unpacked the boxes of good dishes. I have my aunt's dessert plates, too, but we never even think of using them. I used to have such fun getting everything out for a party."

The nodding of agreement started at one end of the room and made the rounds. Then they all talked at once about the family treasures, wedding gifts, heirlooms of silver or china or crystal carefully stashed in cartons in the garage or under the basement stairs. "I don't know why we lugged all that stuff down here when all we do is eat out or have TV dinners. And I used to be a good cook, too."

The committee meeting didn't get back on track until one of the ladies came up with a winning idea: "For this luncheon, we could make it a special affair if each one on the committee would set a table for four or six using those fancy dishes we hauled down here. They don't add anything to our lives sitting in those boxes. Let's share the fun of having nice things!"

Well, that idea caught on like wildfire. The luncheon took on an entirely different tone. "Everyone will want to look at the table settings." And "I should invite my sister from Ocala. She'll love seeing Mother's china all set out." They almost forgot I was going to make a speech, but that didn't matter. These women had found a new joy right in their own cupboards (or cartons).

Later, I had a letter from one of these women saying what you have already anticipated: "We had such a lovely luncheon and so many people enjoyed our old way of entertaining with our own things, I now invite one or two couples over about twice a month or so, to get back some of that fun of early hostess days."

I used to think I was too old to get out the good stuff, set the table, spend most of a day in the kitchen making some chicken dish like Country Captain, which everybody loved so much. Then it hit me. What else has you so busy you can't fix a nice meal and invite in a few guests? In the old days we had to cook something quick to fit in with the family's schedule of ballgames, Scout meetings, and all that. Now they wrestle those problems with their own brood. I have time to spend most of a day getting ready for company and enjoying every minute.

Your town might have different concepts of social life, but here on my turf the days of long-drawn-out cocktail parties have given way to simpler, less-than-lavish small suppers. As we age, that makes sense. Some of our gang has trouble hearing in a crowded room filled with nineteen parallel conversations. Others are uncomfortable standing around holding a glass and a little plate of slippery chips for hours at a time. We get more out of one-on-one or two-on-two sociability. And now that we aren't trying to climb some professional, business, or social ladder, we can relax and enjoy Grandma's soup plates or Aunt Maude's silver service.

Herein lies one of the best cures I know for the boredom of old age. My daughter set me straight on that: "Boredom is 90 percent self-inflicted, Mother. Don't forget that." On a day that seems useless or has no purpose to any of us — widowed, retired, or just plain at loose ends — inviting guests on the spur of the moment might be just the kick you need to feel better about yourself and your world.

Just as the big cocktail soirée seems to have waned, so have the days of long-standing invitations. Those people in the same boat you find yourself in — facing a dreary evening at home again — might be more than available and willing to share a bowl of soup and a game of gin rummy. And go home in time for the 10:00 news. That gives you time to fiddle with the dishes, napkins, and such — almost as much fun as having a doll tea party with Raggedy Ann.

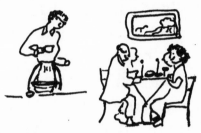

If simplified social life has not hit your neighborhood or your set yet, count yourself lucky enough to play the part of trendsetter. Back in the days of our more forced social pattern, we "couldn't have the Joneses without asking the Smiths and the Thompsons." Now we have single friends who love the chance for an evening of familiar conversation and still-married friends sick of eating dinner and watching "Wheel of Fortune." Home entertaining can be almost atavistic: that which once was necessary for survival becomes a recreation. I cook as well as most chefs, and I love my own leftovers.

A drive to the San Luis Valley of southern

Colorado inspired one of my best Sunday-night supper ideas. That valley grows more potatoes than I had ever seen before in one place. Most are baking potatoes, my favorite. Why not have a supper of baked potatoes with all sorts of toppings, like a pasta bar or an ice-cream-soda fountain?

That idea appealed to my family, but the daughters-in-law suggested that each family bring along a potato-topper. We had creamed dried beef, seasoned sour cream, green Colorado chili, several cheeses, and a crab meat concoction for our potatoes. Tossed salad rounded out the menu, and a good time resulted with little fuss and great sampling going on. The rest of the family and guests have added other creations in more variety since the first potato buffet, which adds to the fun.

Our advanced age provides other forms of entertainment we hadn't often considered in our long-lost youth. How about going for a ride? One day at a time we can discover and learn more about our own territory and enjoy the day instead of moping around about how long it's been since the kids called, or how arthritis seems to have crept into your other knee. No longer chained to school vacation or weekend tripping, we can hit the side roads on a low-traffic day and spend all the time we want exploring old haunts or finding new developments we have previously only read about.

A matter-of-fact sort of older man, who considered leisure time best when snoozing in front of TV news, came to visit me in my condo at Lake George, New York. Now, this old man (in his eighties) had enjoyed the Adirondacks as a child from New York City. He had bragged to me often about the summers he had spent at a camp on Paradox Lake. One day as he settled in for another news-watching snooze just after breakfast, I propositioned him.

"Look, I've seen the exit to Paradox Lake on the Northway not far from here. Let's get in the car — I'll drive and you navigate, and we'll go look for that grand camp of yours."

He hung on the verge of saying, "Oh, that would be too much trouble."

I protested, reminding him of the many times he had told me of the show-biz people who frequented that camp — sons of Broadway producers, and all.

"You even told me that Richard Rodgers and Lorenz Hart were counselors there. You said they wrote shows for the campers to perform. I want to see if anything remains of that famous camp."

He tried to protest again, saying he was too old for such gallivanting around the mountains — besides, he just knew we wouldn't find anything after all these years.

"You were telling me a true story, weren't you?" I tried to look accusing. So finally he gave in. We started for Lake Paradox.

I wish there had been a dozen people with us that day. I wish the whole world could have had the feelings I had, and my friend Sydney had, as we drove around that lake. First he muttered, "There's where the little store was. That's probably all there is to see." Then, one by one, he spotted the tennis courts, the docks, the foundations of some of the cabins, and finally, the old lodge.

Over his objections I parked the car and started through the old fence and waist-high weeds. The building was peeling white paint, torn green shingles on a pitched roof, and a falling-down porch that went all the way around. The floorboards slanted in several directions at once as we carefully made our way to a door hanging open on its hinges. Stepping inside, Sydney's eyes filled with tears. So did mine. The old stage stood there, tattered curtains and all. A trunk or two and some broken chairs had been covered with cobwebs. But right there, on the side of that room, stood a broken-down up-right piano.

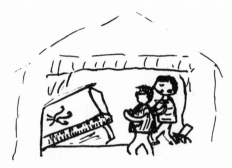

"They did it right there," Sydney said. His eighty-some years seemed to have fallen away. He jumped over some broken boards to stand by the piano.

"Rodgers and Hart. Right here on this piano. That was a long time ago. They were college students, not even regular song-writing partners yet. All of us campers danced and sang on this stage. It seemed bigger then. . . . Our folks came up from the city to see the show. . . . Everyone from the village . . . They came from miles around. . . . We're talking before World War I here . . . I was just a little kid." Sydney's voice, the same voice that had argued successfully before the U.S. Supreme Court, cracked a bit. "We had costumes . . ." He sat down on a broken chair.

We returned to my condo, but when he snored in front of "Wall Street Week" that evening, he had a satisfied smile that made me feel good. We had gone for a ride.

Exploring, whether in search of memories or in pursuit of learning, takes many forms. Consistently popular on cruise ships, shore excursions lead hundreds of vacationers into wider understanding and appreciation of their destinations.

During my most recent lecture-cruise in Alaskan waters, I took advantage of a variety of shore trips. A small airplane over Glacier Bay brought new impressions of those glaciers usually seen from water level. Those babies extend miles back into the mountains. Riding in a jet boat on a river near Haines, I spotted bald eagles in and out of their nests. Humpback whales went into a feeding frenzy just as our small sightseeing boat appeared on the scene. I'd had no idea such a wild happening ever occurred. (Of course, it all happened when I had no camera with me.)

The big event of that cruise turned out to be sport fishing. In July, salmon take over Alaskan waters. (I know that from watching the Discovery Channel.) Catching one of those beauties seemed to me to be impossible for a Colorado housewife. However, my sister, her husband, and I ventured out onto the waters of Sitka and caught enormous salmon, a dozen of those wonderful fish.

The only other time I had been on a fishing trip I had so little luck and so much less interest that I had fished for three days with the same worm. Reeling in those leaping, twisting silver monsters nearly wore me out. But it was worth it, if only to show off the pictures and serve that delicious salmon at home.

Other special adventures? Friends of mine take tours finding covered bridges, natural arches, trails of pioneers. Travel can take many modes from trains to rafts to Model A Fords. Most important: a will to discover and a way to get there.

Many other, smaller adventure rides come to mind: Up in Beulah, Colorado, housewives in a do-something frame of mind picnicked in the cemetery at Rosita. Ghosts of mining camps remain at Rosita, although few buildings now stand there — just a lot of graves. Up there on a clear fall day in the Wet Mountain Valley we discovered the grave of Commodore Stephen Decatur.

What on earth caused a commodore to be buried in a "little mining town in the West"? This picnic discovery started weeks of research into Colorado and naval history, gave us all a new project, and enlivened many conversations before we read the truth about our mysterious commodore. This guy turned out to be a phony. Typical of many men in the last century, he had left at least two families behind, headed for the hills, and actually made quite a name for himself in the gold camps before "retiring" to Rosita.

Other discoveries from going on these rides included Indian artifacts, an old schoolhouse, and several ruins of cabins of early settlers. No boredom in Beulah!

Little children love rides. Grandchildren stop crying for their mothers or stop jumping on the couch when a ride proposal comes along. Cassidy, sort of my great-grandchild, and I took a ride when everyone else had last-minute things to do on Christmas Eve. We admired lights and listened to music on the car stereo.

When the "Nutcracker Suite" came on, three-year-old Cassidy crooked a finger at me. "Now, Oma, this is classical music," she said. Her explanation of the sugar-plum fairies and the snow took half an hour. And I had been complaining about how little today's children are taught! You can learn a lot on a ride. Fondest memories of my own children with their Weaver grandparents almost always include the rides they took. Those little ones need not spend all day at Gram's in front of the TV. As they get older, the roles reverse, but the joy stays.

Role-reversal has taken place in our family (the kids drive, Oma sits in back) on short and long-distance trips. When Jason and Jenny had new drivers' licenses, I needed to bring a car home to Colorado from New York. Driving that distance by myself made no sense when two eager drivers could fly to New York and we'd drive west together. That worked out well. Those youngsters are grown now and married, but we still talk about our experience not shared with the rest of their families. We did Niagara Falls, the bus around the track at Indianapolis, the helicopter in St. Louis, the old homestead in Kansas, and dozens of other places along the way.

One thing about role reversal: When that grandchild takes the wheel, lock your lips (as we used to say in kindergarten). Lay down the basic rules and throttle the temptation to instruct all along the way. That works for me, anyway.

Another pastime popular with some of the oldsters might have started in childhood: collections. Men as well as women really seem to get a kick out of specific items of collectability, particularly small, unusual specimens of certain glassware, artifacts, pottery, and such. I really don't know anyone intent on gathering the big stuff like Hepplewhite highboys, but the small things serve a real purpose in combating boredom.

One man, an old Army buddy of my brother-in-law, has accumulated an interesting number of English wedding bells. Another makes a hobby of finding small turtles of varying design and material. Little turtles typical of the craft of a special region or made of ceramics or native woods add to his travels and serve to remind him of the places he's visited.

Collecting shells rates high on the list of such activities and adds the flexibility of bending over to retrieve an especially beautiful scallop before it disappears with the next wave. My friend Kitty and I made a real study of shells and collecting in Florida one winter. On the beach at Bal Harbor we spent hours bent over, walking miles, picking up all sorts of shells. As a matter of fact, our shell collection grew somewhat out of control.

Every day when we returned to our apartment laden with huge plastic drink cups filled with more specimens of shells than we'd dreamed of, we washed and sorted the entire haul. Finally the old "den mother" instinct overcame us as we looked at every table, every flat surface, covered by shells.

Our next logical move involved the local craft shops and Super Glue. We stuck shells on anything that didn't get out of our way. Baskets, napkin holders, picture frames, mirrors, lampshades, even fly swatters were encrusted with varieties of shells. The boys at the craft shop seemed dubious when we claimed all that glue was for our "shell project." They thought we sniffed the stuff.

Kitty still collects shells, I'm sure. But I have had enough for a while. I have turned my fickle collecting penchant to something more state-of-the-art: videos. Lots of people do that these days.

Aside from the fact that I am deeply devoted to my camcorder (and use those tapes on PBS in southern Colorado), the assortment of tapes for sale in museums, national parks, and other such places tickles me. This makes for collecting that adds more to one's life purpose than a shell-encrusted fly swatter. I had bought Georgia O'Keeffe, Ansel Adams, Seurat, Van Gogh, Cassatt, and other art videos with great glee before I realized I had a collection going.

Now I have added other artists, only one entertainer — Bobby Short — and lots of places. From Costa Rica to Nova Scotia, from Glacier Bay to Cape Cod, we can find an evening's diversion in videos. I have made a practice of finding "place videos" for those long winter nights when TV schedules nothing but mayhem but it doesn't pay to give up and go to bed because I'll wake up before dawn. You can see how such a collection adds more to life than a china cabinet full of demitasse cups. About half of this collection is out on loan to friends and family most of the time.

A similar collection of longer standing — the music of the Big Bands, for example — occupies the time and interest of many oldsters. I found that to be true in a group of Elderhostelers studying the Big Band Era at Arizona Central State College. Records, eight-tracks, tapes, and CDs abound, some truly collectors' items. These serve two purposes since they provide an outlet and focus for the collector as well as reviving the good old days for anyone lucky enough to have (or have access to) such an accumulation of the *really good* music of our generation. Besides, everyone knows the words to sing along.

Here's a suggestion: Send yourself a postcard every day when you vacation. That way you have a collection of pictures of the place and a day-to-day diary complete with dates and notes en route. In an inexpensive scrapbook this makes a fine journal of a trip.

You have probably discovered for yourself what a boon the computer has become to some older folks. For some, just a pastime; for others, a marvelous method of collecting, filing, and organizing anything from family histories to household inventories. Some of my friends have very sophisticated color printers and computers that talk to them. These people learned how to use those machines. Possible. Any diehard oldster who says "I could never do that" is really saying, "I'm too settled in my own rut to explore today's world."

Several years ago I talked with a woman past eighty who had a word processor. She used it to write family letters. "After all," she said, "I want them to know I'm still around, but a separate letter to each of the children, grandchildren, and all the rest took too much time. So now I write one letter, correct the typing, and punch this clever button. . . ."

I remarked about how proud her family must be of her accomplishment. "I don't know if they're proud, but I do know there's something in *my* mailbox every day, and I like that!"

Another thought about how we can entertain ourselves just occurred. Have you gone to a movie or a concert or a play by yourself?

Or are you one of those who missed almost anything that might have been of real interest (museums, shows, and all) because "I didn't have anyone to go with"? Granted, some events are more satisfying with a friend or family member, but don't let going alone mean not going at all. We are reasonably rational about our own safety — and how much protection will an old codger your age be in the face of real danger?

I've decided some women (not you, I hope) refuse to appear anyplace alone because it looks as though they have nobody to go with. None of us care for the thought of looking foolish or unpopular. Forget that. That mindset went out with junior high. If you want to see something, if you dislike the thought of missing something else because Gertrude already had plans to go with Margaret, or because your son-in-law doesn't like classical music, go yourself. In most cases you'll run into someone else doing the same thing. At any rate, you won't be sorry you've missed another show.

Now for more active pastimes. I thoroughly enjoyed watching one couple dancing on a cruise ship. He had retired from Ohio State — history; she looked every bit the dignified wife of a professor. They danced together perfectly. Knew all the steps. Did the right dance to the right music. And obviously enjoyed every dance. No frowns or counting under the breath with these dancers. They twirled around the floor with precision and grace.

"Libby," I said to her, "You and your husband must have enjoyed almost a lifetime dancing together. You're both so at ease and so good! Did you start dancing together in college?"

"Oh, no. We started dancing just four years ago when he retired. Our daughter presented us with a book of coupons for Arthur Murray lessons. Said she didn't want us sitting around the house waiting to be entertained. So Larry and I went to the first lesson and found out he likes dancing as much as I do. We joined a dance group, have new friends and a social life which fits us."

At least a dozen other couples have told me the same story.

Now think about this: For all of those busy years these husbands have gone off to work every day while their wives (you and I) volunteered in all sorts of causes. Today I know more than a dozen men who have discovered for themselves the satisfaction and pleasure of volunteerism. Men in our town have volunteered at the art center, in the travelers' information caboose out on the highway, as a docent at the Pueblo Zoo, in hospital auxiliaries, and as friends of libraries. Frankly, a man's perspective often improves such projects. They tend to talk less and do more. And the women involved appreciate this new approach.

One more aspect of these suggested activities. Don't wear yourself out. We did that. Now our satisfaction comes with discovering something about a painter or a turtle that makes our life fuller. Something to share. Incidentally, I have collected so many kites and art posters that I have turned my garage into a gallery. Oh, the car still fits. I cleared out all of those boxes I've saved and that other trivia, so I have a wondrous time just driving into my own garage. Art and kites? Why not?

Chapter Ten

How in the World?

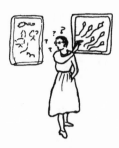

Do you believe in "signs"? Most people stare as if you'd asked about voodoo or hex symbols when asked that question. Well, I sort of believe in signs, as most folks do. Otherwise, why would so many daily newspapers print horoscopes? We all shy away from admitting any dependence on such things, but just let the paper come out one day without the horoscope and the roof caves in. My own belief is casual. If there's a parking place by the Chocolate Factory, that means I'm supposed to have at least one chocolate-dipped apricot before finishing my errands. Since I started this writing business, doors seem to open. People appear in the most unusual circumstances, much more than a "small world" happening. A commonality of experiences that transcends logic — once-in-a-lifetime stuff

— convinces me of the rightness of some activities. Of course, this is all in my head. I am a logical, intelligent woman of good breeding and fine education. I know a fairy story when I hear one. Still, what do you think about some of these signs I care enough to write about? One of the best concerns a happening in San Antonio.

"Who painted this picture? Where did this kite picture come from?" The astonishment must have shown in my voice. As a matter of fact, I could scarcely speak.

Here I stood in an art gallery in San Antonio, Texas, transfixed before a picture of five kites. As far as kites go, these diamond-shaped pastel kites of handmade paper would not attract much attention. Mounted artistically, giving the impression of flying outside a window, the green, blue, yellow, red, and pink kites (with contrasting-color tails curving in an imagined perfect breeze) pleased even the most discerning eye. The sky blue background added to the sense of free flight.

But the picture had more than that. Lettered in between the tails of the floating kites hung the words of a poem:

Skim above me, lively, free,
Ascending as the sunlight beckons
Bait for angels
Wait for me

Then, on one more kite tail, I spotted the name of the poet: *Me*! Right! "Frances Weaver," it said right there, printed in calligraphy clear as day. My kite poem, quoted on this lovely presentation of kites made of hand-done paper mounted and framed in a gallery I'd never seen, in a town I did not know, by an artist of whom I had no knowledge at all. I had shivers up my spine, goosebumps on my arms, and a knot in my stomach. How could such a lovely thing have happened? And how could I just happen to be in this place at this time to see this beauty?

The saleslady smiled at my questions. "Oh, Martha Grant did that. She's been on a paper-making kick, and she loves kites and calligraphy. She found that poem in the *Smithsonian* magazine, so it all came together."

"Did it ever come together!" I fairly shouted. "I'm Frances Weaver! Those lines come from my kite poem!"

Now this dear lady looked stunned. All she could say was, "I'd better call Martha."

I thought she might cry. Even more likely, I felt I might cry, just gazing at that picture. Of course, I bought it. It hangs in a place of honor in my family room, just one more example of the synchronicity that has guided my life for the past fifteen years or more.

Perhaps my perception of events that appear to transcend the realm of mere coincidences has become more keen during these past few years. The first time I shivered over a startling circumstance happened at the very beginning of my writing.

Our kite group of seven (of us) fifty-plus housewives met for lunch one day in March 1977. I had suggested that we should send a report about the joys of kite-flying without children or husbands to a fine newspaper, the *National Observer*. This paper, from Dow Jones, invited readers to write in about their leisure activities. None I had read could compare to the joys of kite-flying. As usually happens with such groups of women friends, I suggested it, so I could jolly well do it. Even though I had no writing experience, the assignment landed on my shoulders alone.

Just as that conversation ended, the phone rang. My husband told me that my dad had just died. He had had a hip replacement and his heart couldn't take it.

Our family had always taken pride in our dad's talent and reputation as a storyteller. Wherever we went, people talked about "John Allison said this . . ." or "John Allison told the best story about . . ." or "Have you heard John Allison's story about . . . ?" I tried to emulate his style or whimsical manner when I finally got around to writing the kite-flying article for the *National Observer*.

Not a writer at all, I sent this piece off on the wrong kind of paper, in the wrong style of type, crusted with correction fluid. The editor responded positively, saying the column about kites would run in his paper, but I would have to wait for a backlog. I told everyone I knew of this great happening in my senior years — a published article in a national newspaper. The bragging turned to embarrassment when the *National Observer* went out of business.

A letter from the editor, Walter Damtoft, apologized for not printing my scraggly effort at journalism, but suggested I should try placing it in a magazine. He thought it would make the grade. Why not? I reasoned. A new avenue of expression, a different look at the world couldn't hurt. So off went letters to magazine editors extolling the wonders and virtues of kite-flying. Rejection slips became a regular part of my new lease on life, but finally I had a positive response from (of all places) *Vogue.*

Now, for a traditional housewife who had never earned a dime in her life, the first check from *Vogue* (eventually I sold four articles and my career as a writer had some basis in fact) thrilled me as I took it out of the envelope. Then thrill turned to chill as I saw the signature on that check: John Allison.

Tears streamed down my cheeks as I stood out by the mailbox. I said under my breath, "O.K., Dad, here we go." Contemplating the entire series of events leading up to the signature baffles me.

Had the newspaper printed the piece, I would have spent the rest of my days boasting that I had written an article for the *National Observer*, probably never trying any other writing. So it fell to Leo Lerman, features editor of *Vogue*, to encourage my attempts with more articles about life as I saw it in Beulah, Colorado. From that day forward, things have fallen into place, leading me to sign books at a bookstore attached to an art gallery in San Antonio, Texas, or to another surprise in Beulah.

The kite article appeared in *Vogue* in March 1978. Quite some time after that, after the following Christmas as a matter of fact, John and I had three adopted grandchildren spending the weekend in Beulah. Now, Beulah has a population of 600 or so, a very small town in the mountains near Pueblo. These children attended Catholic school and were used to attending Sunday services, so I took them to the Catholic church in Beulah. Never before had I been inside that church. Usually I attended Episcopal services in Pueblo with my husband.

The young priest, an Englishman, greeted his parishioners before the service with belated Christmas greetings. He had visited his English home for the holidays. "But," he announced, "on my flight returning to the United States, somewhere over Greenland, I had an unusual experience. I asked the stewardess for a magazine. She handed me the only magazine left in the rack, an old issue of *Vogue*. Can you imagine giving a priest of the church *Vogue* magazine? But looking through the magazine, because I had never seen this magazine before, I found an article about Beulah, Colorado, and some women who fly kites here."

I sat frozen in the pew, unable to move. Several people around me smiled, but I felt I'd just caught a high fly ball in left field and had no idea where to throw it. I just stared. Finally I muttered, "O.K., whoever

You are, I get the message."

Of course, one of the children introduced me to the priest, who couldn't believe the series of coincidences, either. At times like that, what I am doing just feels right. I know no better way to say it.

Almost as startling as such incidents as these, the "small world" meetings with an assortment of people have made a difference in my life. You never know who might turn up.

Just last week, a woman stopped me on the street in Vancouver, B.C., to tell me what a good time she had with her granddaughter on a quilting trip. We had met at an Elderhostel in Arizona and she had taken to heart my advice about traveling with one grandchild at a time. That made me feel wonderful, but it reinforces the small-world concept — that we should be on that same street at the same time thousands of miles from our original place of meeting. Oh, well.

In Capetown, South Africa, at least ten years ago, a traveling friend and I enjoyed the unexpected beauty of the place. The gardens and fields astounded us. We had envisioned South Africa to be nothing more than an armed camp. On a motor tour (with a well-spoken driver in a fine new Mercedes) we admired heavily laden vines and a winery as beautiful and well-equipped as any we had seen anywhere. The architecture was typical Cape Dutch, giving the entire layout a storybook quality.

In the entry hall of the main building my friend stopped beside a guest register. "Are you going to sign this register?" he teased. "You know I never do that sort of thing." I probably answered in a haughty voice.

But I did walk over to glance at the register, which I regarded as a typical tourist thing. "Hey, the last person who signed this came from Kansas!" I sputtered. Further perusal of the signatures revealed that the entire page had been signed by visitors from Kansas. Since Kansas holds a special place in my life — my birthplace, my old home grounds — I read each name with great interest.

There, about six names from the bottom, I read "Hilary and Mildred Wentz, Concordia, Kansas." How in the world could there be more than one couple with names like that? Those people belonged in my husband's family! Cousins of his mother!

I recalled seeing buses in the parking lot. "Just wait here!" I went galloping through an astonished crowd of Japanese tourists just arriving, and reached the parking lot in time to ask the last man boarding the bus, "Is this the bus from Kansas?"

The man studied me for a minute. "Well," he grinned, "the folks on this bus come from Kansas, but we didn't come all the way on this bus."

I ignored his little joke and asked, "Where can I find Hilary Wentz?"

In the three years since John had died, I had not seen these cousins of his, but we greeted each other with open arms there in a parking lot in South Africa, remarking, of course, about "Isn't it a small world?" I haven't seen them since.

Another cousin story fits here. Just preparing to go to my first writers' conference at Santa Barbara, I had a call from my cousin Barbara. Now, this cousin lives in Pueblo and she has spent most of her life telling me how much older and smarter she is than I. This call fit that category (although lately Barbara has claimed to have a Teflon brain — nothing sticks to it).

"Now, Frances, when you get to Santa Barbara I want you to contact my husband's cousin. Such a lovely lady. You really should know her. She lives right there in Santa Barbara. Her name is Trudy Piersall. Trudy Piersall." She repeated the name a dozen times, it seemed. Then she said, "You can remember that name because it sounds so much like 'umbrella.' " Did I say Teflon brain? "Piersall" sounds like "umbrella"? Oh, Barbara connected "Piersall" with "parasol," I reasoned.

Needless to say, the conference of writers, the excitement of listening to famous authors, the entire experience of that Santa Barbara Writers' Conference, wiped out any intention of calling anyone's husband's cousin, no matter how charming.

Two years later I thrilled to every moment of a Lindblad trip to the Swedish Archipelago. Helsinki to Stockholm, actually, on the small vessel *Polaris*. What an experience, and what an opportunity to learn more about the wonders of Scandinavia. Mr. Lindblad himself (a real Swede) accompanied this trip. With a Scandinavian crew, food, and waterways, nothing could have been more delightful.

However, one day in an outdoor museum, I suddenly tired. Even my face felt worn out from smiling so much. Spotting a picnic table, I gave myself a moment just to sit and enjoy the scenery. An obviously American woman sat across, also resting.

"Isn't this a beautiful place?" I said, settling down.

"Yes," she said, looking at the tall pines, calm waters, and glorious islands making a scene that reminded me of a too-real paint-by-numbers picture. "It reminds me of my home," she added.

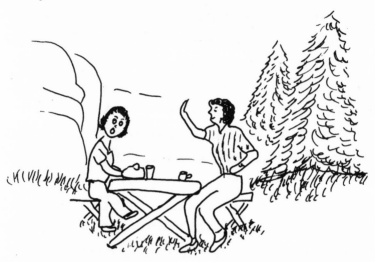

"Where do you live?"

"Santa Barbara, California."

Now I really paid attention to her. "How nice. I love Santa Barbara. Go there every year for the writers' conference." That impressed me more than her.

She felt the need to be polite, I suppose. "And where do you live?" Routine exchange for travelers.

"I live in Colorado."

"Oh. I have a cousin who is a banker in Colorado."

I must have stared. No, this can't — But I said it anyway: "And your name is Trudy Piersall."

Well, she almost fell off that bench. She

gasped, waved her hands in frustration, checked to see if she wore a nametag, and finally said, "How could you possibly know my name is Trudy Piersall, sitting here, total stranger, in the Swedish Archipelago? How could you know that?"

"Simple. It sounds so much like umbrella."

Of course, I explained about Barbara, whom she knew well enough to understand the unusual connection of words, and we spent happy times together on the rest of the trip. Barbara had told me the truth: Trudy Piersall had great charm.

That story makes me laugh. This next one makes me cry.

This same sort of happening took place in Seattle. The Women's University Club, a wonderful group, had invited me to speak for one of its gatherings. Delighted, I went to Seattle for the first time for a real visit to the city.

My book *Where Do Grandmothers Come From?* had just come from the printer. The leading bookstore of the area, Elliott Bay Book Store, had sold enough of my *The Girls with the Grandmother Faces* that I felt comfortable introducing the new book to them while in town. Book in hand, I walked down the hill, awed by the beauty of Seattle.

At the front desk of this marvelous old bookstore, I asked to see the buyer. The girl behind that big old desk gave me a warm smile, phoned for a buyer, and returned to tell me that no buyer could be located in the store at the moment.

I hesitated, certainly not as self-confident as I had felt walking down that long hill. But I showed her my book anyway, with a limp explanation that she interrupted: "Oh. You can leave that book with me. I'll see that he gets it. It's O.K." She grinned. "I know you."

"No. You don't know me. You can't know me. I've never been in your bookstore before. I've never even been much in Seattle before. You must be mistaken. You don't know me."

"Oh, yes, I do. You saved my mother's life."

I'll tell the truth. I almost burst into tears. I almost wet my pants. I mumbled something about, "How in the world could I do that?"

"My dad died six months ago. My mom had a terrible time. She just couldn't do anything. She could hardly get out of bed. I had heard about the *Grandmother Faces* book so I gave it to her. She read it, raved about it, and now she's just fine. You saved her life."

We hugged. I thanked her profusely and left, totally shaken to the core. When I started writing, my goal consisted of spreading the word about the options and opportunities I had discovered open to me in these later years. I had not meant to be a serious contributor to someone's life.

Now, I know very well that girl's mother would eventually have saved her own life, but for my efforts to have served as a vehicle toward her reawakening to the rapture of being alive has to count among the greatest thrills of this life of writing, speaking, and caring about the plight of some older women. No wonder I'm not as old as I used to be!

Chapter Eleven

Elsewhere

A wonderfully well-spoken anthropologist who lectured on board the *Crystal Symphony*, Dr. Fred Levine of Palomar College in San Marcos, California, has set the tone for this chapter on travel — a large part of our senior lives.

Listening to Fred Levine, the realization hit me: He's saying what I've been thinking better than I have said it myself:

For a brief time we have all chosen to give up the routines of our lives.

We have opted to set aside the stability and certainty of the usual.

We've left the security of our domesticity, locked the front doors behind us, and we have tentatively and cautiously stepped into the unknown.

We have set ourselves in motion.

We are here together as travelers, and this is a rare and wonderful opportunity for each of us.

Like many before us we are on a voyage — one not only of sights, sounds and smells, but rather a journey — a journey in which the stage is set for a change, for a transformation of ourselves in this world of transformation — in this ocean of changes. This is a chance for a rare participation of discovery and enlightenment, for a new perception of what it means to be alive. At its best it is an opportunity to be awakened — a means of setting ourselves free.

Travel, near or far, afoot or on horseback (as we used to say in Kansas long ago), does carry this meaning for me. A means of setting myself free to learn, to enjoy, to appreciate the rest of our world, past and present.

On the news this morning the reporter talked for some time about a fire raging out of control in Las Animas County, near here. "Luckily," he said, "the fire blew across the canyon of the ancient dinosaur tracks."

Ancient dinosaur tracks? Near here? What canyon? In my forty years of living in Pueblo, nobody I know has mentioned those tracks.

I'd better get out and see them before another fire comes along.

I might learn more about early Colorado. To me, a journey to La Junta to find that canyon will set me free again to roam unknown territory hoping to see tracks of dinosaurs but also traces of early men — flint chips, arrowheads, scrapers. Not that archeology has that much importance to me, but discovery for myself does. I'll bet I can find a couple of old ladies to go along, too — especially if we have lunch.

On one Pacific cruise we called at Rarotonga, one of the Cook Islands. On this, my first venture into that great reach of the South Pacific, I determined I'd see whatever — people, places, and things. A driver waiting on the dock promised to show my friend and me all of the wonders of this island. (As a matter of fact, the first wonder to me was finding such a small piece of land in so much water!)

Black Rock, the grandest sight on Rarotonga, turned out to be just that — a black rock from which a few people seemed to enjoy diving. I took my video camera down to the edge for a closer look. Scrambling carefully back to the cab, I was met by our laconic driver. "You come my island wrong time."

Wondering what bloomed in the spring, I countered, "What time would be better to come here?"

"When you were young."

I laughed, even though he had no intention of making a joke. I did not bother to explain to him, however, that long song and dance about having time to see the world when we get older. I doubt many people on that island live to my age, so I must have seemed astonishingly old.

Different folks have different ways. We need to remember that and be more aware. The more we understand lifestyles, the more we can assess for ourselves the evening news of conflicts around the world or here in our own space. That awareness, to me, represents the primary reason to "set aside the stability and certainty of the usual."

My traveling friend, Walker Pierce, explores a lot, learns a lot, wherever she is. In a museum in Hong Kong, Walker dropped some books she was carrying and retrieved them without any assistance from the guards and other persons standing around.

"They never even offered. Just turned their backs," she reported later.

Her anthropologist husband explained. "They did not want to embarrass you. The Chinese people ignore whatever appears to be clumsy as a courtesy."

I didn't know that. Walker didn't know that. But we both now understood why the waiters all turned away in Chinese restaurants while we struggled with chopsticks.

The same sort of revelation happens in tripping around our own country. Some everyday occurrence in Atlanta might be unheard of in Minneapolis. We in southern Colorado have little in common with our northern statemates. Nobody who hasn't been there can appreciate Kansas. And so it goes.

We owe it to ourselves to "set ourselves in motion." The next time an announcement crosses your desk concerning a museum outing, a library reading, a community-college class about the people of the Argentine Pampas or the Wounded Knee Reservation; the next time an Elderhostel catalog turns up with a study group for the lighthouses of Maine or the Superstition Mountains of Arizona, give it some thought. That might be just what you need to set yourself free on a voyage of discovery and enlightenment.

When you get home and open that front door, you should be smarter than you were when you left home. At least, we all should know more about the world around us because of our travels. To me, this basic fact shared with grandchildren makes sense in several ways. First of all, you can impress that kid with the fact that Old Granny can still learn.

Most important, you can add to the youngsters' own fund of information broadening their own horizons. In this day of two working parents, grandparents often can fill the gap at vacation time. I thought about this when Betty Yaeger told me about the trip to Crow Canyon she and John will be taking this summer with two grandsons. Those two boys, cousins, will never forget these days of digging in the ruins of the Anasazi in southwest Colorado. They will feel for themselves the wonder of uncovering a painted shard of pottery perhaps a thousand years old. They will also get the fun of learning in a nonschool setting surrounded by others as intent about this archeological heyday as they are.

Lasting, memorable, life-enhancing experiences? How about this one? Rotarians have invited me to speak many times, in a variety of settings. Rotary International, a fine, far-reaching service organization, has a wider outlook of the world in which we live than do most of us.

In Fairbanks, Alaska, my secretary/friend and I attended a district conference of Rotary. "District 5010 covers a lot of territory," our hostess informed us. Well, so does Alaska, I thought. Then she continued: "Our district includes Siberia."

Siberia? Judy and I stared. "People have come all the way from Siberia to Fairbanks for a Rotary meeting?"

This local Rotarian grinned at me. "Closer than Colorado."

During our days at that conference we met and talked to more Siberians than I had ever dreamed of. To a man (woman) they smiled, bowed slightly, and seemed right at home with their American counterparts. Yet their very presence added a dimension to the sessions I had never felt before — the scope of the Rotary philosophy and challenge to ourselves now pervaded the entire world if it reached all the way into the vast Siberian wasteland. Rotary — and I — had come a long way.

The wonder of it all, "a new perception of what it means to be alive," came during the banquet. There in an ordinary college cafeteria seated with three Siberian women who had become our good friends, the *a cappella* singing of the Sharmove Vocal Ensemble, "Rotary's Russian Peace Ensemble," captivated all of us with Russian music ranging from soft romantic sounds to playful folk songs and sombre patriotism.

When they broke out with Broadway showtunes and American favorites, the crowd hit the ceiling. Suddenly, quietly, they started one more number. In the hush of unbelievably beautiful harmonies the accented words began: "O give me a home where the buffalo roam . . ." The state song of Kansas. That hokey old sing-along tune sounded more like a hymn, almost a prayer.

Tears streamed down my face. How could this happen? A Kansas-bred "girl" way up here in Alaska mesmerized by a fantastic group of Russians singing "Home on the Range."

No matter how far we travel, we are never far from home.

More specific travel advice? You don't need advice from me. Travel-advising now ranks as one of the major writing fields of the world. Travel and tourism have almost outstripped eating as a major national pastime. Entire bookstores concern themselves only with travel. Spending half a day in a travel bookstore satisfies the need for inspiration and triggers the curiosity.

Everyone from the Smithsonian to AAA

produces splendid magazines devoted entirely to travel. They line the shelves of your library or cover your friends' coffeetables, just waiting to be read. Regional cookbooks fill in the gaps when we want to know more about life anywhere. Television programming, like the Discovery Channel and National Geographic presentations, exudes information, although sometimes I tire of watching big animals chase little animals and eat them.

In other words, one good look around the reading material available in your own hometown brings the world to your fingertips. Then your "journey in which the stage is set for a change" has already begun.

One more related thought just occurred. In a fine, slick magazine, I read with interest a well-written article about resorts in Fiji. The writer raved on and on about the architecture and furnishings of the cottages, the amenities of the central lodge, the beautiful sunsets, and the crashing waves on the sand.

Then, just as I turned the last page, he complained that these Fijians did not serve *real* maple syrup with his pancakes. Needless to say, I did not finish reading the article. You know why. I know why. We want real maple syrup, we go to Vermont or upstate New York or our local supermarket. Having real maple syrup on our pancakes would be the last reason to go to Fiji. Anyone who expects the best of his own world when going halfway around the globe has missed the entire point of traveling.

I'll bet anthropologist Fred Levine never asked for real maple syrup in Fiji and neither did his talented wife, Nancy. And neither will you or I, next time we venture forth and "tentatively and cautiously step into the unknown."

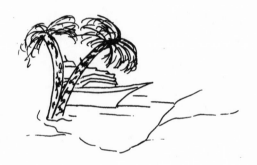

Chapter Twelve

Publishing? You?

"Have you any idea how many books 2,000 is? How many boxes? How many pages?"

Those words from the husband of one of my college friends shook me just a little, but too late to change my mind about self-publishing a collection of my columns. I had been introduced to some of the basics of publishing by helping with a new literary magazine at Adirondack Community College. I had also heard enough speeches by mightier-than-thou editors and agents to know nobody else would put out a collection of columns by an aging unknown. (At that point I dared not refer to myself as a writer.)

Basically, the message from those of the hardback world who deigned to speak to budding authors at all sounded like that song Bob Hope sang in a long-ago movie (about love and marriage): "You can't have one without the other." No agent, no publisher, and vice versa.

Yet my audience for the columns asked for back issues and extra copies. No way would I set the publishing world on its ear, but I could risk enough money and faith in myself to give it a try.

One small incident actually made the ultimate decision for me. Trusting our own decisions had come to my attention as one of the difficulties faced by older women like me. I had needed a different car for quite a while. Driving down the streets of Glens Falls, New York, I passed the Chrysler dealership. In the display window I spotted the first I had seen of the Chrysler LeBaron convertibles. Wood sides. Tan top. Dark-brown body. Slick wheels. Marvelous.

Instead of trying to recall the practical reasons for choosing a car (as John had always done), I simply said to myself, "Who's buying this car, Frances? Who's gonna drive it?" I turned right in to that dealership.

To the young man in the showroom I said, "You've got my car over there!"

"We've been waiting for you!" he replied.

I drove out of the place thrilled silly about that car. After all, I had never chosen a car for myself. Sixty years to get to this wondrous feeling. That dear little car had a Bill

Blass interior of brown leather. The top went up and down with the push of a button. A kind and gentle voice reminded me to buckle the seatbelt or turn off the headlights. (I named it "Walter P.," since Walter P. Chrysler came from Kansas.) "My cup overfloweth" described my feelings perfectly.

Standing in the driveway of the condominium complex on the shores of beautiful Lake George, New York, as Walter and I drove in, my neighbor scowled. I started to say "frowned," but Don looked madder than that. Without any of the expected pleasantries, he growled, "Can you tell me what on earth possessed you to buy *that* car?"

Astonished, I stood a minute and then just blurted out, "I bought this car because I looked all around this lake and I didn't see anyone who was going to buy it for me."

Don walked away in disgust. For one brief moment I felt sorry for that smart-aleck remark. Then it occurred to me: *That's the way your life is now, Frances. No matter what you decide to buy or do, you can look all the way around the lake and nobody's gonna do it for you. Whether you write more columns, publish a book, get along with your family, make the money last your lifetime, remain a contributing member of society. Look all the way around the lake, Frances. Nobody's doing it for you.*

That attitude has served as my foundation. I had some money from John, but he left almost everything in trust to go to our children or to care for me in dire straits. I also had some properties my dad had provided, but not a fortune. I decided to invest whatever I could in myself. That's right, myself. I could create a challenging, rewarding life on my own by spending money on making writing an actual career. My portfolio would be my published work. The return on the money would be a useful, productive life until senility or the ravages of age took over.

John Updike strengthened this determination to "write it out" when he spoke at the State University of New York in Albany several years ago. My good friend Genevieve and I went to his lecture on creativity. Said Updike (more or less), "Creativity demands recognition of what we have already stored in our heads, discovery of our own genre, and an audience." Translating that to my own future, it became clear to me that I could write columns — but where could I find the audience?

Sending several pieces I had written for my college classes to the editors of the *Pueblo*

Chieftain solved that problem. Columnists don't get paid royally, but the audience would be there if I wrote well enough, and that started the ball rolling. Eventually my work appeared weekly in six small newspapers. The income didn't amount to much, but the effect on my life and my writing mattered more. Once I had started writing columns, my awareness grew in direct proportion to the number of words I produced.

During my ten years as a columnist for the *Saratogian* and the *Chieftain*, plus small papers in the Adirondacks and Colorado Springs, my subject matter ran the gamut from sunrises in Tuscany to the havoc created in our world by Doctor Spock, from changes in China to a visit with my fourth-grade teacher. During those years I read little of other columnists, particularly not Erma Bombeck. Although I admired her work, the last thing I wanted was to have anyone think I copied her or her ideas. My own favorite columns, which please me the most, I have included in four self-published books. Here are some samples.

About fiftieth high school reunions, I asked questions:

Have you started your diet?

Begun planning your wardrobe?

Decided to care at all?

I can face facts.

My fiftieth has arrived. I can take it.

I just hope the May Queen shows
up fat.

Our class agent asked for suggestions
for the banquet program. Usually
everyone stands up and brags about
their grandchildren and a prize is given
to the classmate traveling the greatest
distance for this event. I have submitted
a suggestion for the banquet program, a
spell-down trivia quiz about the old
home town. You might find this useful
for your own reunion:

Who was the mayor during our
senior year?

Who ran the bakery?

How many morticians in town?

Did they all rent out folding chairs?

Who starred on the football team?

How often did the town whistle blow?

What was the principal's nickname?

What did we call him behind his back?

Which English teacher had denture breath?

Lists of questions often made a pretty good column. After a confrontation with a self-important widower who had devised a questionnaire for panting, breathless women eager to snag him into marriage, I wrote a list of questions we women should ask any prospective husband or housemate:

Do you like casseroles? Brunches? Eating out?

Do you object to pantyhose on a towel rack?

Have you ever folded sheets?

What do you feed your dog?

Where does he sleep?

Will you eat leftovers? Omelets?
Chinese food?

Did your first wife bake cookies?
Make pasta? Jelly?

Is your mother still living? Near here?

Do you believe in household
budgets? Balanced checkbooks?

How long do you keep magazines?

Do you like Glenn Miller? Long
walks? Museums?

I've decided to settle for a questionnaire
for gigolos. That would be much
simpler. Only a couple of questions
would suffice.

In desperation, I wrote about the lack of
personal service in today's world. I called
this "Where Is He, the Man with the Star?"
In part, I moaned:

Remember those lively, virile, attractive
men who used to sing on Milton Berle's
TV show?

> We're the men from Texaco!
> We work from Maine to Mexico!

Or,

> You can trust your car
> To the man who wears the star!

They're as hard to find these days as a real flying horse at a Mobil station or a live tiger leaping out of someone's tank. One surly individual to read the computers and write up the credit cards and sell Milky Ways is the entire sales and service force. God help you if your engine sounds funny or if the dome light won't go off!

Once in a great while I wrote about famous people. Barbara Bush commanded my attention with her commencement address to Wellesley graduates, so I columnized her, although I'm sure she never saw it.

> Boy, am I proud of her! Barbara Bush doesn't know it yet, but her commencement speech at Wellesley sent chills up my spine, brought tears to my eyes, and hope to my troubled spirit.

Most of us have recognized our First Lady as a woman living by traditional standards. Her value system has to be a lot like mine — her evaluation of herself and her role as a woman and a mother, I mean. What I failed to appreciate earlier was made perfectly clear from that speaker's platform in Massachusetts. At long last the women of my age — women who grew up believing we have a special niche to fill, a preordained role to play that is our own — women like me have the finest, most articulate spokesman we have had in years.

And there are millions of us.

Quotations from that speech will long endure:

"The future of America does not depend on what goes on in the White House. It depends upon what happens in *your* house."

Barbara's reference to old age was poignant and equally well stated:

"At the end of your life you will never regret not having passed one more test, not winning one more verdict or closing one more deal. You will regret time not spent with a husband, a child, a friend, or a parent."

One of her most telling remarks struck me:

"It's not baby-sitting when it's your kid."

Keeping in mind my primary audience, older folks, I have had a tendency, once in a while, to preach. Come to think of it, I still do. This column I called "Creativity Counts."

The "voice from afar" spoke to me again last week. Not often do I get those messages, but once in a while the truth hits with the force of the spoken word. Particularly words I hadn't thought of myself. You know how that goes. All of a sudden you hear yourself saying, "Oh, yeah!" — and meaning it.

No world-shaking communication caught my attention, just a friendly voice saying, "Good for you, Frances. Your life looks really fine in these senior years. But then you always did have a knack with leftovers."

Looking back on these past years of my own life, I can see now the use I have found for leftovers. What leftovers? Just like the celery sticks and the extra chicken, I recognize now that I had stores of energy, curiosity, places I wanted to go, books I'd not taken time to read, subjects I'd never had a chance to study — anthropology, for instance.

It has come to me gradually that any woman who's kept a family on an even keel, survived den-motherhood, and organized fund drives can most assuredly use those same skills in fashioning for herself a life filled with interest for herself and others. Just as she could dump the rice and the chicken together, add a bit of curry powder, the leftover pineapple, and the ever-present can of mushroom soup and have rave reviews for her inventive cookery, so she can mix some old skills with old and new interests and convince her world she's able to fend for herself even when the hair grays and the upper arms tend to sag a lot. (Note: I apologize for that last sentence. It's a dilly!)

On the other hand, if we leave the leftovers in the refrigerator, they'll wither and mold and nobody will care.

My personal favorite column without doubt I called "At Last, Someone to Watch

Over Me." That one told my readers about my new Chrysler.

There's a new man in my life. We've been going around for several months now but I don't even know his name. I call him "Walter P." He hangs out somewhere behind the dashboard of my new talking Chrysler. I've never known a man so helpful, attentive or courteous.

Walter P. cares about me. He reminds me to fasten my seat belt. He tells me when I'm about to run out of gas. He's careful about my headlights being left on. He never lets me walk away without taking my keys with me.

When Walter P. is happy, he says, "All systems are functioning."

A man like that is enough to gladden the heart of any woman. Sometimes when I'm driving alone, feeling a bit lonely, I slow down and open the door just to hear his voice. When he says, "A door is ajar," it brightens my day. I'm pretty sure it is he who turns on the interior lights when I start to get in and who finds FM stations when I'm driving across Iowa. He's a nice guy. I'm lucky to have such a man in my life.

One of my earliest columns still tickles me: "The Disruptive Casting Agency." I had complained to my friend Dell Byrne about a loudmouth who interrupted a writing class at the Smithsonian. This guy made all of us a little crazy. From Dell's response I wrote the following:

"That man came from the Disruptive Casting Agency. I have one of those jerks in my craft class, telling the teacher how to do everything. Last week there was one of their women at my supermarket. She kept running back up the aisles for little things and couldn't find her coupons in her twelve-pound purse. They're all over. It's big business."

It's true. I'm sure of that. Somewhere out there is an office where abrasive people report for work every morning. A brawny woman in a Cecil B. DeMille outfit waves a riding crop and assigns jobs. "Whitsworth, you go on the historic preservation tour and talk about your ancestors." Stuff like that.

You'll find them everywhere. Remember the homey-looking woman whose kids had runny noses and ran wild while she loudly diagnosed every

149

other kid in the pediatrician's waiting room? Or the man with the trumpet voice explaining the menu in the Chinese restaurant? Child stars from the agency are labeled "gifted" and are sent off to drive each other crazy.

Now that your awareness has been aroused you'll be able to identify more and more of these operatives. I'll bet I could get a job there myself.

I've written about penmanship, since I majored in push-pulls (penmanship exercises from my grade-school years). Airports interest me, just considering what some archeologist will find that's worth pondering. The way women handle splitting the check after lunch has been mentioned more than once. Travel makes up a good part of my anthology, particularly the adventure that my friend the professor and I had on a topless beach in Greece. (*We* were overdressed.)

To anyone who asks me about self-publishing, my answer never varies: "It's the only way to start." A plug here for Dan Poynter, the Santa Barbara man who led me along the path. Dan discovered self-publishing for himself and now "poynts" the way for fledglings like me. The nuts and bolts of choosing a printer, an editor, a cover artist, plus the crucial marketing and promotion, all were discussed in a workshop.

Almost anyone who has published his or her own work will rave about the satisfaction in choosing your own printer, paper, typeface, cover material and art, and so forth. Promotion and distribution follow. I made a lot of mistakes and missteps until I learned from Dan Poynter. Until the workshop, I thought I needed to sell through bookstores. Not true. Nontraditional marketing sells lots of books. (I have sold thousands of books through speeches, hospital auxiliaries, gift shops, and mail orders.)

How do we start? First of all: Unless you believe fully and passionately in your subject, *don't bother.* With a sincere desire to "spread your word" no matter what your subject, you can find an audience and a buying public. I recount here my own experience, and I know many others who have followed this path with success and satisfaction.

One of my classmates, Regina Porter, had business experience, which I lacked. Regina also had time on her hands and lots of energy. With her help we made me into a cottage industry. Regina carefully studied local newspapers in upstate New York for notices of appropriate meetings (retired teachers, senior singles, and so forth), then called and offered me as a free program, saying we would also have books for sale with the profits contributed to the good works of their group. Just about two months of that approach set the ball rolling. Since that time ten years ago, word-of-mouth references have kept me busier than I ever dreamed.

When Regina's husband's health deteriorated, she had to quit Midlife Musings Publishing, as we had named me. Another, much younger classmate, Judy Madison, took her place. From that time to this, Judy has scheduled and arranged more than a hundred speeches a year, she has helped me publish eight books, and she has handled shipping and mailing that would make the Government Printing Office weak by comparison.

Back home in Colorado, my children and grandchildren have taken an active part in my projects from the beginning. Chris and his wife Mary have helped with the bookkeeping. My financial acumen has driven them nearly wild at times. Allison has arranged speaking dates for me in Houston. Judy and Sherry, the wives of my two other sons, have taken an active interest in promotion in outlying areas and have been more than supportive in my around-home activities. Each of my children's families has visited me in New York. The solidarity has been a major affirmation of my own efforts.

Certainly my sisters have played a major role. After all, they are pictured on the cover of *The Girls with the Grandmother Faces*. It's pretty much a family affair.

Do you see what I am saying here? *I could not have done this by myself.* What started out to be a few magazine articles and a way to make more of my senior years has grown gradually into a lifestyle I never anticipated or intended. We have just let one door open at a time. To me that describes the essence of self-publishing.

After fifteen years of proving my own worth to myself and my ever-supportive family, my agent and friend Elizabeth Pomada approached major publishers with *Grandmother Faces*. Interviews with the editors of big-name publishers in New York convinced me even more of the validity — the universality — of the subject of affirmative aging. Editors complimented me about the book but spent most of the interview time telling me about their mothers!

Now I'm so hooked on both subjects, old folks and self-publishing, I'm convinced that if someday publishers don't want one of my books, I'll publish it myself.

I just said we have let one door open at a time. That astonished me more than it might surprise you. My audiences have grown from groups of a dozen or so seniors in upstate New York to nationwide audiences including Rotary. I now act as spokesperson for remarkably wonderful continuing-care retirement residences all over the country. My PBS "filler" called "Elsewhere" has had good reception wherever it is shown, and I enjoy doing it with my own video camera. Most of all, I am seeing the world as I could not afford to otherwise by lecturing on Crystal Cruises around the world.

Just one door at a time led me into all this.

Just because I looked all the way around the lake.

Looking around the lake for several years brought me to climactic events — particularly the publication of my (personal) bestseller, *The Girls with the Grandmother Faces*, by Hyperion, a part of the Disney organization.

Hyperion publicists arranged a legendary book tour for me in March 1996. By now you probably have the impression that whatever happens in my life these days surprises me. Right. Never in my wildest imagination had I envisioned myself on one of those coast-to-coast book tours we hear famous authors talk about on the "Today" show or with Oprah Winfrey. The prospect of my appearing at bookstores, at TV stations, and in newspapers all over the country would not have crossed my mind. No list of "I want to be . . ." in my entire life so far would have included such a remote possibility. Yet there I went.

A remarkably efficient young woman, Samantha Miller, had arranged flights, hotels, bookstores, media contacts, and book-tour escorts for twenty-one cities in twenty-three days (I think). I felt exhilarated, secure. But some authors I had heard or read complained about such a grinding schedule, such a wearing experience.

I had read Barbara Kingsolver's account of her tour in her fine collection of essays, *High Tide in Tucson*. She claimed, "My friends think I'm seeing the U.S.A., but that isn't strictly the case. I'm seeing the inside of bookstores, TV studios, radio stations, newspaper offices, and . . . hotel rooms." When days began to blur, Kingsolver started a series of postcards to sort events, places, persons as her tour progressed. "Not that I'm complaining . . . I vow to feel grateful," she continued.

Before Day 3, Cleveland, I recognized for myself the need for some written record. Neither a diarist nor a journal-keeper, I decided to write this tour up as an epic poem. An old-fashioned epic poem. Like "The Rime of the Ancient Mariner" or "Canterbury Tales," neither of which made much sense to me in high school. But poetry these days has no rhyme and little reason. That would suit my purpose. After a few days of thinking about this, I launched the poem project. I bought a sturdy sketch pad (heavier paper) and scribbled in airports, on planes, and in hotel rooms late at night.

This worked fine for me. As I added more and more lines and pages, I could appreciate the word choices necessitated by poetry and could see how my mood swings were reflected in the way I wrote. If it rhymed, so what? If it did not rhyme or had no regular rhythm that descibed my day as well as the words could, that was fine, too. I rewrote very little, feeling the first impressions had more validity for the book-tour account than a revised and edited better piece of work would have.

At home in Colorado, I transcribed the entire thirty pages and read it aloud to my family. Poetry should always be read aloud, even poetry as bad as mine. To my surprise and delight, they not only liked the poem, they asked for copies. After making a few deletions, I have included that poem in this book — not because of the worth of the work but because of its importance in this life that I'm hereby describing as "not as old as I used to be." Not in my forties, fifties, or even sixties would I have felt free to write and share this.

The Grande Tour, 1996 Style

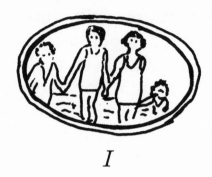

I

It's taken a week
Just to get up the nerve
To start this great epic —
With vigor and verve.
(*Whatever the hell that is!*)
It started in Saratoga
Right where it all began
Warm feelings, good turnout
And old friends on hand.
(*Already I worried about three weeks
    to go!*)
The Albany bookstore
Did not bode well.
Nobody showed up
Would these next weeks be hell?
(*A trainman in Albany brightened
    our day —*
"Aren't you Fran Weaver?"
What a nice thing to say!)

The cab at Penn Station
Fancy Regency Hotel
But dumped at the corner
Pulled our own bags in — Oh, well
(*Why did I expect a red carpet at 11 P.M.?*)
But the next day the limo
With Samantha in charge
'Twas the Nile in Man-
    hattan
I lounged in my barge
(*As Judy sat beaming on a jumpseat!*)
Then —
The green room, the wardrobe,
The make-up — real fine
They all loved my haircut
Said my clothes were divine
(*Sweater, skirt and scarf, new image*)
I sat on the couch next to Joe
As I waited
His friendliness greater than
Anticipated
(*Recognizable by the bald head!*)
Joe Garagiola — big as life
Twice as smart
We bantered and giggled
Felt good — What a start
(*Can I ever forget his line, "I can't take 'yes'*
    for an answer!")
Called from the green room
And in the back door

"Just sit right here . . ."
Lights, people and more
(*Is this big-time TV? One light, one chair
   at a time!*)
I sat and I waited
To meet Bryant Gumbel —
We shook hands, he sat down
The cameras were lighted
He asked questions, I answered
Not really delighted
But just as he finished —
"Dismissed" if you will —
I put in one more line
I can see his face still:
He stared, then he grinned
Then he laughed right out loud —
"The bird or the statue"
And boy was I proud!
That came out of nowhere
From the back of my head
But Gumbel looked humble
A warm human being
Instead of a robot just doing his job
Like a Wimbledon player
After one fantastic lob.
(*Well, I had to rhyme something somewhere!*)
After the show back to Joe
Still effusive
"Don't be modest. How were you?"
"Great" was my answer

Concise and conclusive.
I must have been right
People raved 'bout the show
So in my book of memories
That's the one with the glow.
(*Now I'm appearing regularly on "Today,"
once a month!*)

II

On went the day then
Interviews and lunch
(*Italian, near Skippy's*)
Then another performance
With the CNN bunch
I sat by myself
On a stool with a mike
An earpiece to hear by
No person in sight
But a monitor near by
But I shouldn't look at it
Just straight at the lens
Of a dead-black big camera
Now where were my friends?
(*I guess it worked O.K. They let me
talk a lot.*)

III

Right after CNN to D.C. we flew
To Hotel Sofitel
Which none of us knew
(*Not even Samantha, who booked it!*)
That was O.K. — A great
Young man, Dan,
Provided needed info and
Generally ran
Interference for us as we
Went through the day
AARP radio; Voice of America
And others I talked to
You'd think I'd bore me
But that didn't happen
Each interview differed
I spent all day rappin'
With one and another
'Til time came at last
(*After tea at Hillwood, yet*)
For the Smithsonian Speech
Good God what a blast!
The room filled with people
I stared as they came —
Then I started to speak
And it happened the same
As it has for the past several years:
They all soaked up my message
With laughter and tears

162

Could I have felt better?
Not on your life
Have I done it yet, Weaver?
Are you proud of your wife?
(*Sally Councill and friends, Leo Kasun,*
Sue Somebody, Norman's wife,
and Aunt Kath, yet!)

IV

Now farewell to Judy
At Dulles, no less
What a happy time we'd had —
She knows she's the best
Friend and cohort
An old gal ever had.
Just thinking about her
Makes this old heart glad
(*Terrible line, but I needed something!*)
Let's see — after D.C., the balloon
   really rose
To Cleveland, Chicago, Minneapolis.
   Those
Cities in order on Samantha's list
Fell into place. Began to exist
As a series of interviews,
   tapings and stores:
Shelves filled with books
Voices warm with laughter

163

As I talked about Walter, kids, kites,
    then after
I signed each first name of one,
    then another
And ran for the next plane
Evening flights — limos ready
What a trip this will be
If I keep my hand steady
On each plane germs lurk
Filling the air
To Cleveland, to Chicago, to Tampa
Everywhere
I've caught all they blow at me
Each flight in turn;
Now we've reached a hiatus
The airlines and I
I give back their same germs
Every time that I fly.
I sneeze, cough, and strangle
From take-off to landing
Returning those Airline Germs
    of long standing
(One added surprise in the midst of it all:
The Lutheran Librarians. What
    more can I say?
They're my friends forever — That's
    truly their way.)

V

A note about each town
Which I hit this week
Is surely in order
They've allowed me to speak
On radio, in print and in stores
Surely Ma Perkins could ask for
  no more.
And a page about tour escorts
Before pushing on
These people do great things
I could not get along
Without Dan, Tip, and Marilyn
Not to skip Mary Lou
Each appointment, each desire,
Each taped interview
Comes under their umbrella
They are prompt, exact and smart
They know every station, all addresses
  by heart.
They only do book tours
So meet interesting guests
But with an unknown like me
They seem more of a jest!
The magic word "Disney"
Pervades all my stays
The penthouse in Chicago
For a couple of days
At no extra charge

All was covered by Walt
Including the cashews I consumed
   from the vault.
Just a couple of taxis I've paid for
That's all . . .
When this tour is ended
I'll be in for a fall
Back to reality
One day at a time
But thanks to *that* program
I've earned it! It's mine!
I think of it daily
One town to another
(Without my sobriety
Where would I be?
No chance to discover
The world I now see!)
I sag between airports
I lag after stops
Yet perk up when crowds gather
In bookstores and shops
A weekend in Tampa
Which airport I love
Brought instant revival
Get back on the move
Let's talk about that:
An experience grand
My Florida sojourn
Three days, maybe four,
Brought time with old friends

Ides, Jurons and more
On Monday the Rayfiels
And pals from the ship
Take a deep breath, Frances,
You're losing your grip!
In every bookstore
More chairs they needed
As I prayed for a crowd
And with caution proceeded —
They laughed at the right times
"His brother was worse . . ."
They smiled and they nodded
At my dumb simple verse.

VI

I've never felt older
Never more stressed
Than in Miami airport
May Tampa be blessed!
But that night the crowd
    gathered
In the bookstore again
This one crammed with bookshelves
And my next speech began:
One after another
One flight every night
On to Oklahoma City
What a wonderful sight

Lu Garrison worked her magic
The lunch crowd, impressed,
Bought books, ate and giggled
Who *needs* a rest?
Instead I kept going
From pillar to post
Bollinger's Book Shop
Was that evening's host.
A full sit-down dinner
Lasagna and all
With a speech and some questions
What a treat to recall!
Then I chased off to Denver
DIA — as if that mattered
I headed for Big Time
The world's finest: *Tattered*!
An overflow crowd
Kate, Cy, Tom and Jill
Phyllis Ekiss, Matt and Sherry
What more for a thrill?
Chinook was as friendly
As I needed it to be
But I must backtrack here
I missed something, you see . . .
My day in Denver
Was not much to crow about
No radio, TV
No one I could know about
But one kick of the day
On South Colorado

The escort's new car
A Beetle got in our way.
A small interruption
But what could I say?
Then Kate Miller for dinner
The restaurant atop Tattered
Is really a winner.
(Back to Chinook)
Sister Middy showed up
I loved it, of course
Sam's sister came also
And that was great fun
She had so much young energy
She'll have us all on the run!
We had a fine time
A presentable crowd
The saleswoman thanked us
For laughing out loud.

VII

Pueblo sent me tumbling
Back to earth with a bump
Sarah's not well — she's hurting
I feel like a chump
For taking my own life
So seriously now
That I've shut out the others
Feel a stranger somehow.

VIII

Now comes Arizona
Warm — thank God for that
Colorado was colder
Than a well-digger's hat
(*Whatever that means*)
MM came to Tucson
One helluva drive
But we had a great visit
Sisters learn to survive
In Tucson more interviews
And a fine escort, too
(*To be included in my final report*)
The bookstore at Tucson
Barnes & Noble? Borders? Who knows?
Was an absolute thrill
As a book signing goes . . .
We had dined with old friends
Jones, Sharkey their names
The food was just awful
But they were not to blame
And all was forgotten
As a special crowd gathered
For a short talk and questions
And signing. I blathered
My way through the first part
So thrilled there to see
Luke, John and Charlie
Who meant my world to me

Back in Upstate, a long time ago
And here they show up
My world took on a glow
Then there were Mackin's
from Cripple Creek, yet
And Janet Quarles' daughter
You'd think she'd forget!
Old Wick hugged me tight,
And Marie from the first days
With regards for Regina.
The whole thing was a maze
Of folks from my yesterdays
Here to confirm
Their joy in my progress
I raved in return.
The best was dear Charlie
Who's been such a dear friend
We hugged and we kissed
And we laughed at each other
My cup runneth over
There's just no other way
To say one evening in Tucson
Made a very special day.
On the drive up to Phoenix
MM and I chatted non-stop
Caught up. Exchanged stories.
Watched a comet.
(*I value the times*
We can pay total attention to each other.)

The big deal in Phoenix
We were signing at Borders
Goes back to first pages
But I'll put it in order
Of the way it all happened
Steps one, two and three,
With Joe Garagiola, his daughter and me.
A "wired" group of women
Effusive, just charming
Their enthusiasm struck me
Just short of alarming
Appeared at the table
I'd given no speech
They crowded around
They all talked at once
"Our writing instructor . . ."
I heard, then "showed us your book"
"She sent us to see you"
(From Elderhostel)
By then I was hooked.
"Her dad told her about you . . ."
So who's her old man?
Baseball player — TV star
Imagine if you can
My astonished reaction
When they named the
      same man
From my "Today" attraction
Joe Garagiola! What could be better?
He not only liked my book

He promoted it
With his daughter
And Elderhostel
Even now as I write
My smile gets much wider
I'm as high as a kite!

IX

Off to Portland
The scene was routine
A few old friends — new ones —
But the store was a shock:
A feminist bookstore
In a real crummy block.
But a few of them
     showed up
Much to my surprise
I made no pretense
Couldn't tell any lies
About being liberated
Which I surely am not
But it was a new experience
So well worth the shot.

I'm sorry to say it:
Seattle was worst
All the good times before that
Slipped into reverse

No car out at SeaTac
Though one had been hired
No hotel reservation
Should Shirley be fired?
She just gave me bad info
Perhaps *she* was wired!
But round about midnight
I'm not ready to battle for
A hotel room of my own
In the streets of Seattle, for
To my plane-weary bones
That's too much of a chore
"Just any old room . . ."
I bravely implored
Well, it worked out just fine
With an elegant suite
At 240 a night!
Mickey Mouse won't repeat
Mistakes like this one
It's really a honey
I had a fine room,
But Mickey lost money!
As if the hotel botch was awful
The airport came close
To disaster — United delayed
I'd miss a DIA connection
A fate worse than death
If I had to spend time in that laughable zoo
But good old Delta saved me
I knew they'd come through.

X

Now it's all over
Repercussions abound
I'll soon head for New York
To see what can be found
At the end of this rainbow
This "trip" so enticing
It's like having no cake
The whole world is icing!

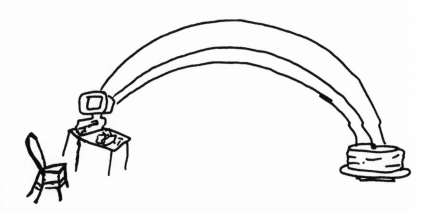

Chapter Thirteen

Granny! How You've Changed!

Had anyone even suggested to my grandmother that in her seventies she might be
writing a chapter about grandmothering for
a new book, she would have laughed and
said, "Oh, pshaw, why would I do that?"

In Gram's day grandmothers sat on
porches visiting with neighbors, made
chicken potpie for the church suppers, wres-
tled with the Maytag wringer every Monday
morning, darned, wrote letters, listened to
the radio once in a while, and sent the kids
to play in the attic on rainy days. At least,
my grandmother lived like that. Did yours?

We read and hear a lot these days about
the changing role of grandparents. Some
"experts" seem to think they've just discovered the phenomenon of creative roles some
grandparents play in the lives of their families. Do you recall the Norman Rockwell

painting of a small boy and his grandmother at a table in a bus stop diner? Travel with grandkids might be more widespread in the '90s just because we oldies live longer. But a thoughtful, caring grandmother has not changed in any real degree. The world has changed around us and we make the most of it. We do more of some things and less of others in comparison with preceding generations. Thus has the family always worked.

My guess is that more analyzing of all of us — our goals, our expectations, our responses — must give some do-gooder the impression he's found a new trend or even a radical breakthrough. My contention — first voiced in my book *Where Do Grandmothers Come From?* — remains firm: Grandmothers come from other grandmothers. We pattern ourselves after role models, good and bad. No authority on behavioral science needs to tell any woman cuddling her first grandinfant that she's in for a special relationship. We women know that. The way we express, nurture, and enjoy that relationship adjusts to the current lifestyle of the family. In other words, let's get down to basics here: We go with the flow.

In the really olden days, Grandma probably helped the actual delivery of the new baby out behind a bush, then guarded the infant from snakes and prairie dogs while the parents went out hunting and gathering. As the child grew, that gram could see to it that he or she learned how to plant corn or catch bugs. Might even have admired juvenile graffiti on the cliff walls on rainy days.

Centuries and generations later, those grandmothers spent time with little girls showing them how to stitch doll quilts or braid their own hair while busy mothers worked in the fields. At the same time, Grandpa taught the boys how to bring in a mess of rabbits with a home-made bow and arrow.

Do you agree? Grandparenting can never be called "new." We've done this forever, but the demands of the day give each succeeding generation of "grandies" new responsibilities, different challenges, and certainly wider satisfaction within the family.

A warm, appreciative grandmother told me about her five-year-old who had just graduated from nursery school. (Did we say our world has changed?) This angelic child in her cap and gown explained to her "Mumsie" what her school required for

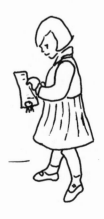

graduation: "First we had to learn our computers. We learned to write our daddy's name and where we live and our phone number and if we make any mistakes it's just delete, delete, delete, and do it again!"

My sister Mary in Arizona sends videos of herself to grandkids in Denver to establish recognition and communication between visits. The children think their gram is a TV personality, I suppose. When they get older they can reciprocate with videos of their own. Or by that time they might all be using the Internet.

Lifestyles have changed so drastically in the past few years that for some of us keeping up with a child's world resembles a journey into outer space. Thomas Edison's folks must have felt the same way.

Time spent with the youngest generation must invariably result in the strongest affection and the most pleasant memories. That statement comes from personal analysis. I cannot recall any present I ever received from any grandparent. Can you? They must have given my sisters and me all sorts of fine things, but no memory comes. Times spent "helping" Grandmother Allison run the wet clothes through the wringer of that Maytag, days of hiding from our mothers as we cousins darted around Granddad Jensen's orange grove while he grinned at our game, nights of listening to Grandmother snore at the other end of the sleeping porch — those I remember. (We put on shows and she clapped.)

When I ask my own children for memories of grandparents, they seem to have the same responsive feelings. Each spoke first of going for a ride. With their Weaver grandparents, they spent happy days in the backseat of the old Ford on country roads. Joe Weaver drove that car as if it had an automatic shift. Once down their alley and out onto Republican Street in Concordia, Kansas, Joe shoved that baby into second and never touched the gearshift again.

Joe always took our boys to get haircuts on their Kansas visits without parents. I thought the haircuts were terrible, but the boys had a wonderful time.

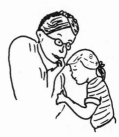

My daughter Allison just turned fifty. Asked about her grandmother Vesta, Allison's eyes mist: "Vesta could always fix things. Vesta could always make everything all right. I knew when I was little I could depend on Vesta to help me. She made things for me like that purple square dance skirt and doll clothes. She'd sing in the car or whistle. Sometimes she'd just pat my hand."

Wouldn't you love it if one of your grandkids recalled you with that much love? I surely would. Notice the basic: Vesta's attitude, her caring, her time-giving made a difference that has lasted far longer than her life.

Now how do we make such an impact, such an impression of love on our own grandkids in this day of video games, horrifying movies and TV shows, and a constant ranting and raving about the breakdown of the family? The best way we know how is one day at a time. That's how we've always done it.

One big area of opportunity for building strong ties with our grandchildren lies in the fact of so many career mothers. Vacation time for the family once depended only on Dad's time off. Now Mom has work responsibilities as well. Travel has involved grandparents more and more. Coupled with the longer life of the old folks and the enormous energy of some of our senior travelers, kids find tripping around with Gram and Gramp a fun experience.

Again, this vacation with grandparents has not just come on the scene. You probably went someplace with your grandparents, and so did I. Our children traveled even more with our parents. Now grandparent–child vacations have become routine. My dad set the example for the rest of us in vacationing with grandchildren. Dad had no brothers and no sons. His homelife consisted of women. Grandsons enjoyed the greatest of vacations when Dad took all seven (only one was too young to go) in one of the first Dodge motorhomes for an extended drive through Colorado, New Mexico, Arizona, and California. Rumor has it they even went to Mexico, but we mothers never heard the whole story.

Years later, long after Grampy died, we still learn more about the goings-on with that bunch of boys and that trip. Their grandfather left a large portion of his estate to those boys, who are now in their forties — greatly appreciated, but what they talk about still is that journey. Grampy was fun, Grampy was smart, Grampy slept in motels while the boys slept in the motorhome in the parking lot and considered an hour in the motel pool sufficient bathing.

According to the *New York Times*, vacations are becoming a time that far-flung families come together. The newest term is *multigenerational travel.* Soon we will find reams of statistics about the trend. Cruise lines report more family groups than ever before. And not only the Big Red Boat of Disney attracts cruising families. Holland America reports a substantial increase in families of three generations sailing together. On Crystal Cruises, the luxury cruise line on which I lecture, we see family groups, and the ship has special "camp counselors" to entertain children during the day plus a special playroom and a video gameroom.

In my own grandparenting I have enjoyed great trips with my second generation. We have spent time, without their parents, building relationships that we find individual and delightful. Best advice: Enjoy vacationing with the grandchildren from about six to college age. Too soon they marry and have jobs and families, and have little time for Grandma's outings.

Now as my grandchildren mature and marry, and as my children anticipate grandchildren of their own, I look back at my most active years with younger offspring. Those days when Whitney insisted he could stay up until 9:30 because he was gifted. That's before he made the deal with his mother that still holds today: Whitney brought water from a well on a camping trip so his mother could shampoo her hair. In return, Whit does not have to eat three-bean salad for the rest of his life. Next month Whit will begin his law career in one of the most prestigious firms in all of Texas. No wonder!

How can I forget a grandson like Jason, so polite and concerned for my feelings as he asked, "Next time you make this delicious jelly, Oma, could we just drink it?" With his master's degree from Stanford, Jason passes along his kind ways to his students at Sequoia High School in Redwood City, California.

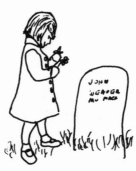

Miss Sarah, the tyke who gave me the name for my book *The Girls with the Grandmother Faces*, etched memories into all of us. I learned from Sarah about taking time to explain life's events to very young children. Only four years old, Sarah went with some of her cousins and brothers to see the grave of their grandfather. Largely ignored by the bigger kids, Sarah stunned all of us by asking, "Is this where Pal is died?" We nodded. "Well, it's no wonder," Sarah said. "He can't get any air down there."

The other grandchildren and I have had good times, too. They came into the family already half-grown by virtue of second marriages, so I missed their smallest years but we have made up for lost time, I hope.

My own across-the-street Grandmother Allison loved music. Her favorite song, "When I Grow Too Old to Dream," delighted her when my sister Mary sang it. Those words have been spinning in my head as I have written this chapter. Facing the years past, looking at the fine time I'm having as a grandmother, but more especially facing the future, there's a basic truth there: When I do grow too old to dream, I'll have all this to remember.

Right now I am seventy-two. Lifespans have stretched well beyond these years of mine. Perhaps mine will, too. But I do feel old enough, experienced enough at living, that building memories is a great part of what life is about now. Not just my own memories of family, friends, books, cruises, speeches, the "Today Show," or my little PBS series. I'm talking lasting memories in the lives of people I've touched.

Shared memories are the basis for all of my carrying-on with all of these grandkids, my sisters, and the rest of my family. When I have been with Sarah in Greece or with Jenny and Jason at Niagara Falls, almost all of that has been learning, sharing what we alone have in the midst of the family. I have no doubt there will be times after I die when the younger family members will recall unpleasant or difficult times with me. I'm not trying to be Mary Poppins or Ma Perkins. Not even Tinker Bell.

More than any other recollection, I hope to be thought of as one person who added something positive to their lives.

This has a lot to do with love, but very little to do with obligation. Years ago I heard an old lady say, "Write anything you want on my tombstone. Just don't say, 'She meant well.' "

Like Grandmother's song, that rings in my head a lot. None of the fun, the pleasure I have enjoyed with my family, has come from a sense of "I ought to do something nice for these people because we're related." Instead, the trips, the games, have been as much for my own amusement as for theirs. I just hoped to choose the right venture for mixed generations. After all, I'll be too old to dream long before they reach that stage.

Back in grade school we played a game, "Pass it on!" Remember? It occurs to me those could serve as code words for grandparents. Pass it on. All the good I recall from my own grandmother I have tried to pass along to my grandchildren. Certainly I cannot claim 100 percent success. My grandmother career resembles the rest of my life: sometimes on target, a lot of near-misses. Still, I trust these generations will pass it on.

I can picture Ross and Judy climbing around Mesa Verde with Sarah's sons, or Chris and Mary showing the wonders of the Grand Canyon to one of Andy and Charlie's brood. Or perhaps simply making cookies with a messy, happy little girl of Whitney's will be Allison's joy in grandparenting.

Who knows?

Just pass it on.

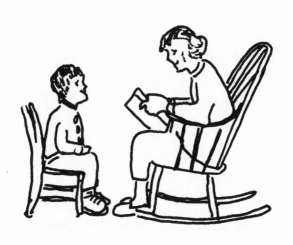

Chapter Fourteen

Today, a Different World

Underlying every bit of advice or observation about aging, we recognize one great truth: We live in a world none of us anticipated. That makes it hard to keep pace in more ways than fax machines and the Internet. Very nearly every aspect of our daily lives has changed. I read someplace, "People born before and after World War II might as well have been born into two different worlds." I believe that, don't you?

This comes up in conversation incessantly. Talk about the good old days invariably turns to, "Families used to take care of the old folks. Grandma moved in. They all got along. Now parents get shoved off to a home for old geezers." From that point the subject expands.

My own opinion — supported by many wise people I know — makes sense, at least to me. Back in the days of our youth Grandma fit into the household of the next generation and enjoyed being there because she had a real part in daily life. It was Granny who darned the socks, washed the dishes, ironed the napkins, mashed the potatoes, baked the cookies, hemmed the dresses, discussed everyday affairs with her daughter, cut paper dolls with granddaughters, made herself useful.

How can you or I feel useful in a home filled with push-button laundry, paper napkins, and kids hooked on video games? Grandmothers in our day made rich chocolate cakes or peanut-butter cookies that tasted marvelous with an ice-cold glass of whole milk. Today's children think home-made cookies come from the Pillsbury Dough Boy. They'd choke on whole milk. These youngsters already fuss about salt, cholesterol, and too much sugar while they feast on Twinkies and diet Coke.

In our homes as we grew up, dishwashing often involved the family singing over the sink. For one of us to move in with our children expecting the same sort of fellowship while switching each other with damp tea towels makes sense only to us. The microwave and dishwasher quite literally replaced Grandma years ago. We have to learn to live with that — to become today's grand-parents just as our younger generations have become today's families. Who have you seen cutting the tops off the carrots lately?

It all boils down to Today's Fact: Today's family households do not require enough "housework" to make an older, healthy, active woman or man feel productive, useful, or appreciated. And that's a fact. We can't even help the kids with their homework unless we know as much as they do about computers.

This sad state of affairs cannot be blamed on ungrateful offspring. They feel the responsibility and want to do the right thing. The changing world has made the biggest difference in our need to feel needed.

Living as my grandmother did, I might gripe about spending all day Monday up to my elbows in suds in the basement, but I'd know I had done something by the end of the day. The fragrance of sun-dried sheets and piles of dazzling white underwear would reward the labors of the day and I'd take all the credit. How do I replace that satisfaction in my own life?

For years I have claimed that living alone works for older women. One old lady I admired said she'd "never had the refrigerator or the bathroom all to herself in seventy years," so she was not about to give that up now. Most of the women I know, and some of the men, find smaller quarters more sensible than the four-bedroom family homes with a lawn to mow, gutters to clean, furnace filters to replace, windows to wash, and shrubs to trim. In townhouse living, most of that burden belongs to the home association. All we need to do is dust.

In the ever-growing number of retirement communities offering lifetime care, we don't even have to do that. This makes even more sense for couples and single oldsters alike. Convenience and security count, of course, plus the services provided on a varying scale up to assisted living and intensive care. But to me the importance of the sociability of such retirement centers ranks high on the list of advantages.

When it comes right down to it, these facilities (the well-planned, realistically financed ones) allow us to keep one foot in each of our worlds: the old one associating with people who understand the magic of the Big Bands or recall with us the days of gas rationing, and the new world of computers and videos, if we care to try.

The other day I watched with fascination as a man on television explained how much information now can be accessed through home computers. Encyclopedias, magazines, books, all sorts of data-collecting material can be ours in our own home if we just know which button to push. Most challenging: This man described the abundance of information available not for college students, not for professors in great universities. He addressed this discourse to us, the old folks.

How many of your friends have announced, "Why should I know about computers? My broker and my banker use computers. What do I need with such a contraption? I have no need for such rubbish." My friends have talked that way. But this man pointed out one very important point. Even a person in a wheelchair can keep in touch with the outside world by e-mail. Even an incapacitated oldster can find information, recreation, and amusement. In other words, we can remain independent thinkers and doers with computer literacy.

Just think about it. I haven't made the big step to the Internet yet, but I have long valued the wonders of word processing. Now — as soon as I have time — the entire world can be at my fingertips if I only take the time to learn how to access it. One of these days I might depend on computer-based knowledge. My family will be proud.

So there we find one answer to the question, "What do I do with all of this time on my hands now that I have so few daily chores? How do I feel useful? How do I amuse myself without needing the family to take me out to dinner or suggest a Sunday ride?" Perhaps, just perhaps, computers fill the bill for you. Many oldsters I know have set up genealogy programs in their computers and have gathered their family histories that way. Others have hooked into travel or cooking or history programs. Think how that widens our world. A shrinking sphere of ideas means only one thing: a self-atrophying brain.

One more thought about the role of older women in the household: While writing this, the sights and sounds of the South Pacific have surrounded me because of a lecture/cruise. Yesterday in Saigon I saw old women squatting on the grubby decks of houseboats washing pots and pans with water from the river. You can imagine my thoughts: There but for the grace of God go I. Perhaps life at my age in my country needs some adjustment, but I'm not squatting by the river washing the dishes. That would just ruin my knees!

Chapter Fifteen

Hang onto the Rapture

Joseph Campbell said it: "We seek not so much the meaning of life as to hang onto the rapture of being alive." Does he mention "easy" or "fun"? No. A much stronger word, an almost uncomfortable word instead — the *rapture* of being *alive*.

Notice he doesn't say anything about someone else handing us this rapture. We seek it. It's up to us. Well within our grasp lies the rapture of being alive, but our antennae must pick up the vibrations that direct us to that goal.

What has so set me off on this near-tirade that I have gotten up early to write about it? Why does this subject cast itself in my mind as the ideal penultimate — there's that word again! — chapter for this book? Thanks to a fellow passenger, who will have no idea she's being thanked, I see more clearly than ever the message I have been striving for years to convey.

Let me tell you about this woman, whose name I don't know but to whom I shall be forever grateful. We sat at lunch where conversation ranges from trivial to casual.

"I don't go to the lectures on this ship. Just what do you lecture about?" Her tone of voice told me no answer would interest her, let alone please her.

"Generally, I speak about the options and advantages of being old." Other voices at the table chimed in with words like "wonderful," "hysterical," "inspiring," which she ignored. The way she looked through me would have frightened some ladies I know.

The staring contests of seventh grade came to mind. I smiled, ever the optimist.

"Don't be stupid," she snarled. "There's no advantage to being old. Here I am, still around. My husband has died. My children have died. Why am I left here? What is there in this world for me to be happy about? Why? Why? Why?"

At the moment I had no answer for her. In that social setting no polite, concise reply entered my mind. Grasping at straws, I said, "The least we can do as widows is try to be someone our husbands and family would be proud of."

Her astonished look served better than any words. That look of astonishment brought me to this word processor before breakfast. Why? (Now *I'm* asking.) In a world filled with people less fortunate, millions or billions of people starving or suffering, that woman sat here on an elegant ship, with all of the luxuries and amenities known west of any given point, and whined. Obviously, all of her worldly goods did not suffice. Why? She had no sense of the real worth of herself.

Money can't buy it. No one sells it with a designer dress or plastic surgery. A fancy car cannot bring the appreciation of ourselves and what we can contribute just by being alive. That rapture starts with an assessment of ourselves, our potential, and the possibility of some small change(s) that will reclaim our purpose in life. In other words, recycle ourselves.

Just the word *old* takes more of a beating than any other word in the language today. For a word its size, *old* creates even more bad images than does *age* or *die*. We hate that word *old*.

Good "old" speaks of fine wine or oft-repeated family stories or long-standing friendships or the satin finish of fine antique furniture. Good "old" speaks of the Big Bands or Marlene Dietrich or Big Little

Books or Will Rogers or Dionne quintuplet paper dolls.

Bad "old" evokes backaches, weak bladders, and sagging pantyhose. You should never need them, but let me give you Fran Weaver's four sure-fire rules for looking old:

First, never comb the back of your hair.

Second, wear the same bright red lipstick you loved in college.

Third, never fail to mention your rotten son-in-law.

Fourth, whine. No matter what, whine.

The choice is with each of us: We can achieve our own definition of *old*. Personally, I'd rather be "old" with some pride, some justification for my pragmatic attitudes — and most of all, some sensitivity for others my age.

More than any other aspect of life in my seventies, I want my family to be proud of me. That does not mean I need to set the world on fire or become famous. It means I need to reach out to the rest of my world with understanding, real care, and a determination to cope with my own problems and my own future. I see that as an achievable goal at any age, but more important as we ourselves age.

Sam Levinson put it this way: "God never promised Mama happy." That line has stuck in my head since I read his fine book, *In One Era and Out the Other*. Look for that book. My own copy is long lost. "Happy" is not a goal. "Contentment" and "serenity" or "satisfaction" apply more to us now.

"But I feel so alone sometimes. My kids are busy with their kids. . . ." We hear that whining over and over. Consider the contrast between being "alone" and being "on our own."

Visualize the difference.

"Alone" raises the image of a sour old hatchet-face watching the soap operas and fuming over the talk shows while the world goes on outside her door.

"On your own" we see an older woman who participates in the world around her and reciprocates with her family and friends on her own special terms. She or he doesn't have to be "on the go" every minute, but every day brings something to look forward to, whether it's line dancing at the senior center or a classic movie at the library.

Old people can benefit from today's new world in ways they might not have considered. I'm a firm believer in some sort of community living. (You've heard that from me many times.) I have also advocated the use of home videos or audiocassette recordings for communication over long distances — a video or audio exchange with your grandchildren in Oregon, for example.

Now picture this: A bunch of old people living in the security, convenience, and sociability of a retirement center. The activities director shows up one day with a simple camcorder for use of residents.

Immediately the challenge is thrown out. "Why don't each of you make a video of your life here in Pleasant Acres here in Kansas City of golfing, the exercise class, or craft session or just visiting with friends? Send it to your grandkids in New Jersey. Invite them to send a video of their school, home, and Little League team for you to share with your friends here." Ask yourself one question: Why not?

The world offers such challenges and opportunities every day: Computers. E-mail. Can't you just see one of your family bragging to the neighbor kids, "My Grandma is on-line. She can't walk too good, but she's great on her computer." Or "Grandpa sends me videos and they're not bad!"

The biggest investment, and for some of

us the most difficult, is ourselves. The greatest reward? A finer, deeper sense of our own
worth, our own being, our own durability.

Epilogue

Welcome to the Club!

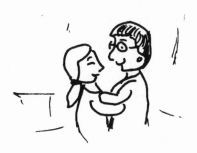

"Oma, what are you doing for dinner? Matt's busy, so I thought I'd pick up some Kentucky Fried for us and come to your house. O.K.?"

"Sure! Thanks!"

What a pleasure, daughters-in-law. Sherry arrived, chicken in hand, distress written all over her face.

"What's wrong? You sounded fine on the phone."

Close to tears, Sherry hugged me — darn near clung to me like a little kid.

"Oh, Oma! The boy at Kentucky Fried gave me a senior discount without even asking!"

Well, I thought, it's finally happened. Just in time to get themselves all settled in their new role as senior mentors and experts of the world before the beginning of a new century, the "boomers" have turned fifty. Such a momentous series of occasions has not taken place in this or any century — not so many people at once all qualifying for an AARP card. The computers at Prudential have buzzed at top speed for months getting ready for the onslaught of half-century birthdays. And this will go on for several years. Our lobby in Washington (whether we participate or even agree) promises to grow to unheard-of numbers.

Other offices, like Elderhostel, and certainly all of the government agencies devoted to complicating the daily lives of anyone who lives to the ripe old age of fifty, can claim backlogs of "work" up to at least 2020 (A.D.).

Just imagine the joy at Social Security. The prospect of this gang's turning sixty has become a reality. "Hire more people! Stuff more stuff into more machines! Close down more local offices! Invent new mysteries in the system to confuse an even larger bunch of old folks! Forget the endlessly busy 800 numbers. We can drive these new oldsters crazy with e-mail and the Internet."

In no time at all, we will begin to read and hear about these "boomers" growing up in a primitive world. Their children will anguish with them over the old days, watching

Howdy Doody on black-and-white, listening to forty-fives until their folks could afford eight-track tapes — those incredible days when nobody had even heard of CD-ROM or Pampers.

They will agonize over being raised on whole milk, sugar, peanut-butter-and-jelly sandwiches, bologna, plain old vitamins with no antioxidants. The worst deprivation, of course, causes even these fifty-year-olds to cry: eating at home — particularly eating hamburger cooked by their mothers.

Some might mention the good old days — hula hoops, poodle skirts, home permanents. And they'll rave on about their old-fashioned parents (us) who thought they ought to be learning to memorize poems and recite times tables.

Although I have not seen statistics to prove my opinion, it has occurred to me that this generation of fifty-plus persons — our children! — constitutes the first generation in the history of the world to have more parents than offspring. Think about that. My children, my sisters' children, my friends' children, all have smaller families than we had. Some have not even replaced themselves on the planet. At the same time, our generation and some even older parents live much longer than parents before us did.

Do you foresee a world top-heavy with old folks? I do. That accounts for my determination that we should all make the most of our later years before these come-lately senior citizens try to take over our world of retirement and love.

I can see it already. These young Turks who have been responsible for changing the way we eat, the music we try to understand, the dress code everywhere, the movies we avoid, the miserable communication on every level, the social standards on which judgments are made, the very air we breathe — they are now set to become just what they accused us of being: cantankerous old goats dead-set against any new ideas.

These are the people who have created the household words Prozac and Spandex. They have made monumental strides for the good of mankind with their health clubs, exercise machines, mountain bikes, and roller blades.

They eat things like algae and seaweed.

They have put gloves on dentists, the rest of us on hold.

They have devised a new lingo — new meanings for "tape," "room," "surf" — and they wonder why we stare. They have computerized everything from bass fishing to home movies.

They claim to have invented sex. Now

they'll invent old age.

Picture this: All of a sudden we shall be inundated with new expertise about grand-parenting. Of course, some of these folks have put off having their first batch of kids so long they are now confronted with high school wrestling tournaments, learners' permits, and menopause at the same time. Some of them will experience the empty nest and feel compelled to instruct the rest of us in coping, naturally.

Will these fifty-year-olds have the same hang-ups about getting old? Will they try as hard as some of our generation does to hang on to the appearance, the image of youth? Will they accept aging as a logical, expected part of life or will they expect to stay "boomers" forever? Will they look upon us as the generation that can show them the way to a satisfying old age, or will we be in their way? Will they appreciate or resent the miracles of modern medicine that have kept their parents alive until their expected inheritance has either been used up by the old folks or doesn't reach their hands until they themselves have no energy left to enjoy being our beneficiaries?

When I started writing about aging and its advantages, I wrote about getting along with adult children. Now those adult children have adult children of their own. I expect advice from them, don't you?

Sooner or later, you or I will meet some fifty-five-year-old who has discovered for herself the options and opportunities of later life. She'll have a disgustingly upbeat attitude, urging every old person west of any given point to get out there and make life count. She'll have a sappy smile and make us laugh. She'll tell old-people jokes. Then she'll announce to us that she's written a book.

Do me a favor, folks. Pat her on the head and tell her it's been done.

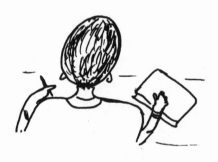

About the Author

Frances Weaver, 72, is a widow with four grown children and eight grandchildren. After the death of her husband in 1980, Frances chose a return to college at age 58 as the vehicle for changing her lifestyle and living as a single woman for the first time in her life. She lectures across the country and runs her own company, Midlife Musings. Frances is the Seniors Editor for NBC's "Today" and the author of eight books, including *The Girls with the Grandmother Faces*. She divides her time between homes in Pueblo, Colorado, and Saratoga Springs, New York, and frequent lecture/cruises aboard Crystal Cruises around the world.

DATE DUE

DEC 2 0 1997	
DEC 27 1997	
DEC 3 0 1997	
JAN 1 4	
JAN 2 7 1998	
FEB - 8 1998	
FEB 1 9 1998	
MAR 3 1998	
MAR 9 - 1998	
MAR 3 0 1998	
APR 3 0 1998	
APR 0 2 2002	

GAYLORD   PRINTED IN U.S.A.